T0099956

THEORISING
in **EVERYDAY**
NURSING
PRACTICE

We'd like to dedicate this book to nurses and nursing students who theorise in practice while delivering excellent care under difficult conditions.

THEORISING
in EVERYDAY
NURSING
PRACTICE

A critical analysis

HELEN ALLAN
KAREN EVANS

Los Angeles | London | New Delhi
Singapore | Washington DC | Melbourne

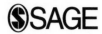

Los Angeles | London | New Delhi
Singapore | Washington DC | Melbourne

SAGE Publications Ltd
1 Oliver's Yard
55 City Road
London EC1Y 1SP

SAGE Publications Inc.
2455 Teller Road
Thousand Oaks, California 91320

SAGE Publications India Pvt Ltd
B 1/I 1 Mohan Cooperative Industrial Area
Mathura Road
New Delhi 110 044

SAGE Publications Asia-Pacific Pte Ltd
3 Church Street
#10-04 Samsung Hub
Singapore 049483

© Helen Allan and Karen Evans 2022

This edition first published 2022

Apart from any fair dealing for the purposes of research or private study, or criticism or review, as permitted under the Copyright, Designs and Patents Act, 1988, this publication may be reproduced, stored or transmitted in any form, or by any means, only with the prior permission in writing of the publishers, or in the case of reprographic reproduction, in accordance with the terms of licences issued by the Copyright Licensing Agency. Enquiries concerning reproduction outside those terms should be sent to the publishers.

Editor: Alex Clabburn
Assistant editor: Ruth Lilly
Production editor: Jessica Masih
Copyeditor: Jane Fricker
Proofreader: Jill Birch
Indexer: Caroline Eley
Marketing manager: Ruslana Khatagova
Cover design: Sheila Tong
Typeset by C&M Digitals (P) Ltd, Chennai, India
Printed in the UK

Library of Congress Control Number: 2021940522

British Library Cataloguing in Publication data

A catalogue record for this book is available from the British Library

ISBN 978-1-5264-6836-9
ISBN 978-1-5264-6835-2 (pbk)
eISBN 978-1-5297-6620-2

At SAGE we take sustainability seriously. Most of our products are printed in the UK using responsibly sourced papers and boards. When we print overseas we ensure sustainable papers are used as measured by the PREPS grading system. We undertake an annual audit to monitor our sustainability.

Contents

About the Authors   vi
Acknowledgements   vii
Foreword from Professor Pam Smith   viii

1   Introduction   1

2   The changing nursing workforce and the emergence
    of nursing knowledge   13

3   Theorising in practice   26

4   The studies   44

5   Theorising in practice through workplace recontextualisation   57

6   Theorising in practice through workplace recontextualisation
    among experienced nurses   81

7   Theorising in practice through learner recontextualisation   102

8   A new relationship between nursing knowledge,
    theory and practice   129

9   Concluding thoughts   145

References   160
Index   175

About the Authors

Helen Allan is a Professor of Nursing at Middlesex University, London, UK. She registered as a nurse in 1979, working for 13 years in acute care. After a BSc in Sociology at the London School of Economics, London University, Helen trained as a nurse teacher and taught social sciences and nursing at Bloomsbury College of Nursing & Midwifery and then at the Royal College of Nursing Institute. Helen completed her PhD in Nursing part-time at Manchester University in 2000. She worked with Professor Pam Smith at the University of Surrey in the Centre for Research in Nursing and Midwifery Education. Helen has held Chairs at the Universities of Surrey, York and since 2014 at Middlesex University.

Helen has worked as a nurse teacher and as a researcher for the last 20 years. She's particularly interested in how nurses learn in clinical practice and the role of emotions in clinical practice and their effect on learning.

Karen Evans is Emeritus Professor of Education at UCL Institute of Education (University College London). She has held professorships and academic leadership positions in the University of London and the University of Surrey, where she directed the Postgraduate Centre for Professional and Adult Learning and was a founder member of the Centre for Research in Nursing and Midwifery Education. Most recently she held the Chair in Education and Lifelong Learning at UCL and served as Head of Lifelong Education and International Development in the Institute of Education, University of London. She is a Fellow of the Academy of Social Sciences and holds Honorary and Visiting Professorships in the United Kingdom, Australia and Latvia.

Karen has worked as a university researcher and teacher for over 40 years. She has interests in professional learning and how development depends fundamentally on multiple forms of knowledge which practitioners continuously develop and put to work in practice.

Acknowledgements

This book forms a part of the legacy of the work of the Centre for Research in Nursing and Midwifery Education at the University of Surrey where studies 1, 2, 3 and 4 were undertaken. The ideas in this book are the result of the research work supported by the Centre.

Helen Allan would like to thank her colleagues at Middlesex University, Sinead Mehigan and Michael Traynor, for being understanding about where her energies have lain during the writing of this book.

Karen Evans would like to thank UCL Institute of Education for its role in providing sustained support for novel ideas and approaches that involve cooperation across institutional, disciplinary and professional boundaries.

Karen and Helen would also like to thank all the research participants and research colleagues in each of the five studies who have contributed to ideas which they have developed in this book.

Foreword

Pam Smith

In their book *Theorising nursing in everyday practice* Helen Allan and Karen Evans bring together the very best of nursing and education scholarship and research to address 'a fundamental conundrum at the heart of nursing'.

Helen Allan Director of the Centre for Research in Nursing and Midwifery Education, University of Surrey (2008 - 2013) and currently Professor of Nursing, Centre for Critical Research in Nursing and Midwifery, Middlesex University and Karen Evans Emerita Professor and former Head of School of Lifelong Learning and International Development at the Institute of Education, University College London bring a wealth of research, education and practice to craft in this original book.

Indeed the role of theory in a practice discipline remains a conundrum not only in nursing but also in other practice disciplines such as education and social work. What is special about nursing however, is the centrality of care and its association with women's work. Allan and Evans spell out from the very beginning that context is everything, from the wider historical and societal issues which shape a profession to the particularities and specificities in producing new knowledge and practice learning.

Helen Allan draws on her own context of learning, teaching and practising nursing to ask questions and set the scene. Helen's personal approach invites readers to reflect on their own experiences of theory and practice to relate and engage with the book's premise that the production of knowledge is a lifelong liminal activity in response to changing environments and relationships.

The context in which I undertook my own research in the 1980s on the emotional labour of nursing bore many similarities to the nursing world described by Helen. Nursing theories, the nursing process and the activities of daily living underpinned nurse education and practice. Student nurse apprentices were influenced by the ever powerful ward sister and taught by nurse tutors often regarded as cut off from the reality of practice and clinical teachers who at best helped support them in the wards.

The world has changed dramatically over the intervening decades. Nursing students are now university undergraduates rather than apprentices and as Helen acutely observes nursing theories have all but disappeared from the curriculum. First mentors, and now practice supervisors, have taken over practice education from ward sisters and clinical teachers. The organisation of healthcare has become financially driven with devastating effects on patient care and safety as revealed by the Francis Inquiry (Mid Staffordshire NHS Foundation Trust Public Inquiry, 2013). In the light of these damming findings one of the Inquiry's major recommendations was that there was an urgent need to improve support for compassionate care within healthcare. The events leading to the Francis Inquiry undermined not only nursing's confidence in itself as the major caring profession but also the public's trust in it. The Covid-19 pandemic has restored much of that confidence and trust in nurses as the doyens of compassionate care.

The book is particularly timely to view these many changes through the lens of 'putting knowledge to work' illustrated through five case studies. These case studies are well chosen to address the contemporary nursing world and the many changes that have taken place over three decades to reconceptualise and re-contextualise nursing learning and practice for the twenty-first century.

The first study investigates leadership for learning by mentors and nurse managers following the post 2000 changes in nurse education including the move from hospital schools of nursing to universities, giving student nurses supernumerary status and an end to apprenticeship style training as NHS employees. The rupture in these traditional relationships, ways of working and learning as a consequence of these changes are not to be underestimated.

The second case study continues the theme of the fallout of change. Here the focus is on the transition of newly qualified nurses as they learn to manage patients and the complexity of managing support workers who were originally introduced to take over the front line care from student nurses.

The third case study is well chosen to highlight the modern health service and the changes in governance and incentives to manage patients with long-term and complex conditions in health and social care. The focus of the study is on interdisciplinary mental health teams and their roles in the community management of patients with long term mental health conditions. This focus on mental health is particularly apt given the urgency of mental health matters highlighted by the pandemic.

The fourth case study is based on Helen's ground breaking doctoral research on developing fertility specialist nursing roles and the holistic care of infertile couples. The particular insights brought to bear in this and case study five is that nurses continue to learn throughout their careers.

Case study five updates the reader on the changing roles of senior nurses based on recent research which investigated the role of commissioning nurses or GBNs (governing body nurses). This study is important because it considers new senior executive nurse roles where commissioning of direct nursing care plays no part in those roles.

These case studies hold the key to why conventional nursing theories did not endure and why a dynamic way of conceptualising and re-contextualising nursing knowledge and theory is required. These case studies demonstrate that nursing and nurses are not homogenous, relationships are not static, and that nursing and nurses are part of the bigger picture reflecting society and the role of women. Ethnicity, race and class are part of this bigger picture, with the pandemic exposing the many inequalities and discrimination experienced by black and ethnic minority communities in general and health care professionals in particular.

The book reconceptualises nursing knowledge around the core concepts of person, health, environment, with a contemporary emphasis on climate change, shaped by social changes and the need for nurses to theorise in their own particular way and style across different workplaces at different stages of their career. I find these ideas just as exciting now as when first heard 'hot off the Press' from Karen and her colleagues, David Guile and Judy Harris, at the Institute of Education (Evans, Guile and Harris 2009). Their innovative research looked at the challenges of integrating theory, practice and work based learning by vocationally orientated learners as they mediated their way between formal and practice knowledge, professional and vocational identities. In this book Helen Allan's ground breaking research on nursing leadership, education and practice puts this approach to the test to show just how apt it is for understanding the multifaceted contexts of learning and practising nursing in the complex and post-pandemic world of the twenty first century.

Four of the case studies featured in the book were undertaken by the Centre for Research in Nursing and Midwifery Education at the University of Surrey. I was privileged to be the second director of the Centre and honoured to be invited to write this foreword. The book makes a major contribution to the Centre's legacy and a fitting tribute to its first Director, Professor Rosemary Pope. It will provide stimulating and thought provoking reading for years to come.

1

Introduction

Chapter objectives

- Introduce theorising in practice
- Present our understanding of contextualising and recontextualising knowledge as the basis of professional learning
- Propose what we see as a false dichotomy between realism (doing) and idealism (thinking) in nursing
- Conclude with an overview of the chapters in this book

Introduction

This book is a collaboration between Helen Allan and Karen Evans, who met while working at the Centre for Research in Nursing and Midwifery Education at the University of Surrey. Helen is a Professor of Nursing at Middlesex University now and Karen is Emeritus Professor of Education and Lifelong Learning at UCL Institute of Education, London. The book grew out of work we did together while Helen was at Surrey University. The book addresses a fundamental conundrum at the heart of nursing: the role of theory in a practice discipline. Our contribution to the debates over theory in nursing is to argue that nurses theorise in practice continuously. We argue that grand theories, models of nursing and mid-range theories do not adequately explain how nurses theorise in practice. Our intention in this book is to show how recontextualisation, reworked in nursing practice, does.

Who's the book for?

This book is written for those who have an understanding of the role of theory in practice disciplines. We don't introduce or discuss nursing theories in any detail. We presume a certain level of knowledge about either education theory or nurse education. We refer to and discuss education theories to develop our argument in the book. This is, of course, exactly what nursing theorists have done to develop their theories of nursing. But we don't intend to introduce yet another theory of nursing.

Unlike other textbooks on nursing theory, we do not intend to describe or discuss nursing theories and apply them to practice as this has been done elsewhere. We refer to several nursing theorists and come back to the role of nursing theories and theorists in nursing in Chapter 8. In writing this book we are building on existing analyses of nursing theories and their application to practice, e.g. McKenna (1997), Murphy and Smith (2013: Vols 1–3). These authors suggest that theories are largely ignored by practising nurses today. They argue that nurses use knowledge, they apply knowledge where it is appropriate and construct their *own* knowledge where the knowledge they have is inappropriate or inadequate. Quite clearly, nursing is theoretical and evidence based! Our premise in this book is that existing grand theories, nursing models and mid-range theories of nursing do not capture nurses' theorising in practice. Therefore, unlike other textbooks on nursing theory, we start from practice by drawing on nurses' descriptions of the knowledge they use in practice. We have captured their descriptions of thinking (theorising) during research interviews and informal conversations as we observe and participate in their practice. During these research encounters nurses as participants were given the opportunity to reflect on their practice in ways which do not occur in ordinary everyday practice as they're too busy.

There are a number of excellent texts which do introduce nursing theory and nursing theorists which we refer to throughout the book.

Introducing theorising in practice

The initial impetus for writing this book arose during fieldwork on a research project into newly qualified (registered) nurses' experiences of their transition from student nurse to staff nurse (Magnusson et al., 2017). The following episode took place during participation observation of student nurses in a hospital trust in England. A *trust* is an organisational unit within the English National Health Service (NHS), generally serving either a geographical area or a specialised function (such as an ambulance service). In any particular location there may be several trusts involved in the different aspects of healthcare for a resident community, e.g. mental health, learning disability, acute care. During a quiet period at the end of the shift, Helen asked a student nurse 'What nursing theory do you use?' She immediately replied:

'Oh I don't know any nursing theories.'

After a while she said, 'We're taught to write up our care using the Trust's (hospital's) values.'

Helen was struck by:

1. Her assertion that she didn't know any nursing theories as a 3rd year student nurse.
2. Her assumption that the values of the NHS hospital trust where she was in placement would guide her nursing reports – that they would stand in place for nursing theory.
3. The way she thought writing ('write up our care') might answer Helen's question about nursing theory. Her view implies that for her, rather than theory helping her to think about the care she gave, theory was more about the care she 'wrote' up, record-keeping if you like.

Helen wondered what shaped her giving of care; she mentioned the trust's values but how did they shape the care she delivered? Was 'writing up her care' the only point at which she *thought* about values and thus in some way, linked thinking and doing?

A few years later, Helen worked with Karen Evans on study 2. And as a result of ongoing research conversations, reflected that in the new BSc programme curriculum at the university where she teaches, there is very little recognisable nursing theory as she recalls teaching nursing theory in the 1990s. Values derived from the UK Department of Health's NHS values (NHS England, 2012, 2016a, 2016b) are taught, but nursing theories as such aren't taught anymore. There's a module called 'scientific knowledge', and another called 'nursing knowledge'; the scientific knowledge module is orientated to introducing the student to evidence-based practice and an understanding of research process. The nursing knowledge module includes the nursing process and focuses particularly on nursing assessment.

This student nurse's experience was very different to Helen's experience in the 1970s when she trained on an apprenticeship, modular training programme. She was introduced to a medical model of care where *nursing care* was tacked onto the medical treatment. This was a similar model to Nightingale's model of teaching probationers in the 19th century (see Chapter 2). The teaching of nursing theories and the nursing process began in the UK in the 1970s. Helen's introduction to nursing theories began in the 1980s as an ICU ward sister studying for her Diploma in Nursing. She was introduced to theory through nursing assessment when she had to assess a patient using a nursing model or theory. She chose Roper, Logan and Tierney (1985). Helen found their Activities of Daily Living (ADL) model helpful in identifying the contribution of nursing to critically ill patients' recovery in general and in describing what nurses were doing for the patient she selected. Of course, it fitted the acutely ill patient as it was based on the biomedical model.

At the same time, she was encouraged by the clinical teacher (who was the link with the School of Nursing) to introduce nursing care plans into the ICU based on a chosen model of nursing. So, she suggested to her colleagues that they introduce Roper, Logan and Tierney's ADL model to the intensive care unit they worked in. Helen was happy to do this because the ICU staff were struggling to justify why they needed qualified nurses with a post-registration certificate in intensive care nursing working in the unit rather than nurses without such a qualification; they were also under pressure to measure their workload and patient dependency. Helen felt (from her own learning on her Diploma course) that using the ADL model care plan would help the staff identify both to their medical colleagues and the hospital managers what the nursing contribution was and therefore what the staffing needs might be.

Introducing the Roper, Logan and Tierney model into practice proved a really difficult project, which met with huge resistance from the nursing staff and dismissive contempt from medical colleagues. But it planted a seed of a thought for her about the potentially unique contribution of nursing to patient care and what knowledge nurses use to underpin their caring practices.

After graduating with a Bachelor's degree in Sociology in 1990, in 1992 Helen taught nursing theory to student nurses studying on the Project 2000 Diploma in Nursing at Bloomsbury College of Nursing and Midwifery. In 1996, at the Royal College of Nursing (RCN), London she taught nursing theories to registered nurses studying for their top-up BSc in Nursing Studies (at the RCN). The nursing theories which made sense and helped her understand what she was observing in clinical practice at the time were caring theories; like Watson (1979, 1988) and Leininger (1981, 2002). Helen continued to believe that caring was fundamental to nursing and this was supported by her empirical observations in her PhD. However, she also began to draw increasingly on social theory to understand nursing and caring practices in fertility nursing.

At the point Helen met the student nurse described above, she had begun to ask herself whether caring continued to be at the heart of nursing (practically) and if not, what relevance all those years of teaching nursing theory had achieved! She also wondered whether nurses do not necessarily think in terms of nursing theory anymore. From a number of studies investigating learning in nursing which are drawn on in this book (see Chapter 4), she has concluded that when offered the chance to reflect on their practice, nurses do think about nursing and the knowledge they use to inform their practice. In her experience, most nurses, irrespective of how distant they may be from frontline (fundamental 'bedside' care), continue to care and to think and thus theorise about caring and their actions as nurses. For some, this is in one-to-one relationships, for others this may be about care for populations. However, when asked about theory, in Helen's experience, most nurses' eyes tend to glaze over.

Of course, thinking about nursing theory is alienating if the theories themselves appear to be removed from one's experiences of practice and if they're imposed on nurses from education or the trust. This is, of course, the way much of nursing theory was introduced in the UK. By the 1980s, nursing theories were introduced to the curriculum and by the 1990s, became even more important partly because of the *new start* nurse educators envisaged with the introduction of the Project 2000 curriculum. We all aspired to disciplinary knowledge to underpin our curricula. Nursing theories seemed the way to achieve that.

Unfortunately, grand theories and nursing models by theorists like Henderson, Peplau, King and Watson were introduced largely uncritically and, frequently, imposed on busy nurses (McKenna, 1997). Busy nurses enthusiastically, and sometimes unenthusiastically, introduced theories into practice, again largely uncritically. This imposition squeezed out theorising in practice and contributed substantially to the antipathy towards nursing theories in British nursing – especially as most of the theories were developed for nursing in an American healthcare context.

Helen's research, spanning 2000–2020, shows that nurses do think theoretically – they just don't necessarily think about nursing theories. By this we mean that nurses think about the reasons why they're caring in particular ways, they articulate to each other in handovers or in case conferences the rationale of what the nursing care is based on, and they think through ethical practice based on their knowledge of ethical theories and intuitive ethical knowing. In other words, they are theorising but not drawing on established theories of nursing (Reed, 2006a; Rolfe, 2006a). Helen now feels her original question to the student nurse was wrong. She should have asked something like:

- How do you make sense of your role in this ward?
- What knowledge do you find most useful?
- Does it help to apply certain theories or knowledge in practice that you've learnt in college?

In that way she could have tapped into the student's active learning and processing of theory. As a result of that interaction with the student nurse and drawing on a range of research projects which have investigated nursing knowledge in one form or another, Helen has moved from asking 'what theory do we use?' to asking:

- What is the role of theory in nursing practice today?
- What knowledge do nurses draw on to inform their practice?
- How do nurses use knowledge?
- How do they conceptualise their practice?
- What place does nursing theory have in current learning and teaching in the 21st century?

This book is a result of all these reflections and conversations with co-researchers over the years and with Karen Evans in particular. We have observed as researchers that nurses are usually ready to reflect when asked why they do what they do in relation to their everyday activities in clinical practice. In doing so, they articulate theory, that is, they draw on a range of different theories or knowledge which seem relevant for their practice and make meaning for them – they theorise or develop knowledge for practice. They may not articulate this meaning every day – they don't have time; but there are (increasingly squeezed) spaces for this thinking to happen or for spaces to be made (Allan, 2011). Thus, we have found that nurses are happy to articulate theory in research interviews. Helen has also found that both registered and student nurses are happy when asked in class to reflect critically on their work and to use and develop knowledgeable practice. Nurses, when given the opportunity, are critical thinkers and theorise.

Therefore, in this book, we aim to show how nurses theorise in practice drawing on research data from a range of clinical settings: general medical and surgical wards, extended, specialist practice in fertility nursing, community mental health nursing, clinical commissioning groups. And in different roles: as newly graduate nurses managing the boundary between nursing and support workers, interdisciplinary working in mental health community roles, in commissioning and as specialist fertility nurses.

Contextualising and recontextualising knowledge as the basis of professional learning

In this book we are concerned with how nurses, through their learning in practice, develop theories of practice. Perhaps they would describe this as nursing theory – perhaps they'd say it was justifying their role or showing the impact of their role.

We argue in this book that their reflections (which we illustrate through research data from a range of projects) are theorising in practice. Like Reed (2006b) and Rolfe (2006b), who argue that nurses produce knowledge in practice, and Avis and Freshwater's approach to critical reflection (2006), we do not describe this thinking or reflection as *applying* theory in or to practice. We have taken a different approach to theorising to Reed, Rolfe and Avis and Freshwater. We draw on Evans et al.'s (2009) ideas around contextualisation and recontextualisation of knowledge as the basis of professional learning. Basically, Evans et al. (2009) argue that we rework knowledge for practice across different settings whether we're engineers, nurses or teachers. Their approach is a way of understanding the theory–practice gap which doesn't reify that (so-called) gap. We explore this further in Chapter 3.

Recontextualisation theory has been used in other vocational learning settings – freelancers in film and TV (Bound et al., 2014, 2015), further education teachers (Loo, 2014), aircraft maintenance engineering (Evans, 2015), camera operators in the film industry (Evans, 2015). This book develops ideas originally set out by Evans et al. (2010) in a special edition of *Nurse Education Today*.

Realism (doing) vs idealism (thinking)

We think there is a continuous tension between realism (the *doing* side of nursing) and idealism (the *thinking* side of nursing) in nursing practice. We believe that this tension is continuously reproduced (and has been for a long time) in nurses' talk about a theory–practice gap. This gap creates a false dichotomy between the doing and the thinking sides of nursing where a circular argument is created. Even talking about the doing side of nursing may be a false dichotomy as doing is thinking in action (Alderson, 2020). As Jackson and Barnett state, 'learning itself is practice. We cannot learn without doing something' (2020: 2).

Consider this quote from the *Delegate study* (detailed below) which shows how the theory–practice gap is reproduced in everyday nursing work within nursing teams. The speaker is a healthcare assistant (HCA):

> Yeah, yeah, I don't think you can learn everything you need to know from books, I think a lot of it is got to be there and experience it and be hands on, there's only so much you can learn out of books. I know you've got to do like your theory which is fair enough but most of it, you can only learn through experience and on the job training because there's certain things you're going to see while you're working that you're never going to read in books.

See how this HCA describes a common denigration of nursing theory in the central point in this extract: (theory) '*is fair enough but most of it (nursing) you can only learn through experience*'. She suggests '*there's certain things you're going to see while you're working that you're never going to read in books*'. So rather than seeing theory and experience (learning in practice) as complementary, as a way to deepen learning, she sees them as antagonistic. So, we prefer to talk about splitting of theory and practice rather than understanding it as a gap; understanding theory–practice as a gap creates a false dichotomy and ignores the thinking in doing. Using the word 'split' instead of gap requires us to consciously think of splitting theory from practice. It reminds us that we are all splitting theory and practice artificially. We explain our discomfort over the tension between doing and thinking by blaming or projecting the blame onto or into someone or something else – it's the lecturers' fault, they've lost contact with practice; it's my mentor's fault, she doesn't nurse according to what I've been taught in college. We continue to believe in something which actually doesn't exist (the theory–practice gap) and we reproduce the gap through our thought as if it exists without thinking about it (the gap) critically. In sociology, we would call this a reification:

> The error of regarding an abstraction as a material thing and attributing causal powers to it – in other words the fallacy of misplaced concreteness. An example would be treating a model or ideal type as if it were a description of a real individual or society. In this case, the error is treating the theory–practice gap as if it really did exist concretely. (*A Dictionary of Sociology* (1998) Oxford: Oxford University Press).

Helen concludes that nurses are pushed into thinking this way partly because they are pressed for time and overwhelmed by competing demands. Partly because current theories used in nursing, e.g. evidence-based practice or nursing as complex interventions, don't account for much of what nurses do. Consequently, there does seem to be a concrete gap. And partly because the older theories of nursing which described caring as a central task of nursing seem outmoded. Nurses' time to deliver care is increasingly circumscribed as their roles become technically complex and caring is devolved to care assistants. However, this doesn't mean that nurses don't care or that their new roles aren't based on the same values or thinking that have shaped nursing practice and education for over a century. Plenty of nurses would disagree with us here (see Bradshaw's [2017] strong response to the Francis Report). They'd cite the Francis Report (2013) and similar scandals of poor nursing as evidence that virtue-based caring has disappeared in the 20th century as a result of changes to nursing education and nursing roles.

However, Helen hasn't seen any abandonment of a caring attitude in her students or in nurses when she talks to them; she *has* observed a lack of caring in practice. We argue in Chapter 2 that this is the fault of a healthcare system which relies on poor staffing and fails to invest in those staff who work in the NHS, as well as the change in nursing responsibilities described above. For Helen and the nurses she's interviewed, nursing is about developing relationships with patients and their families and/or carers to promote health and wellbeing; nursing roles are underpinned by knowledge and values around the person, health, environment, care and self-care, and society. None of the grand theorists' claims that care is at the heart of nursing seem outmoded even 50–70 years after they were written. Helen was heavily influenced by Watson's theory of caring when she studied the caring theorists for her Diploma in Nursing. And this was reinforced and expanded in her PhD when she incorporated concepts from Peplau's (1988) psychodynamic theory of nursing into a practice theory of fertility nursing. Helen would happily adapt Leininger's (1981) maxim that 'caring is the central, unique, dominant and unifying focus of nursing' to 'caring is the central, dominant and unifying focus of nursing which nurses engage with in their work with others to deliver and supervise the delivery of care'. But as Donaldson and Crowley argue (1978), clinical (nursing) practice has always been too narrowly defined for a variety of reasons which we shall explore in Chapter 2. Care and caring are still at the heart of nursing but the delivery of care is much more complex in modern health systems. Professional competency goes beyond that required for delivery of individual, personalised healthcare (Manley et al., 2011). And any profession must be defined by its social relevance and value orientations rather than by its empirical truths which we shall see cannot always be established. This is as true for medicine as it is for other healthcare professions. This relevance is as much local as it is general, i.e. national, and nurses should be free to adapt theories to local practice (Manley et al., 2014; McKenna, 1997).

The evaluation of the *Compassion in Practice (CiP): Nursing, Midwifery and Care Staff: Our Vision and Strategy* undertaken in 2015 (NHS England, 2016a; O'Driscoll et al., 2018a) showed the effect this tension between realism and idealism has on nurses. The purpose of the evaluation was to identify the outcomes of various programmes of work, values and behaviours that have been developed as a result of the strategy and how these have influenced and/or supported nurses, midwives and care staff's experiences of delivering care. There was a clear difference in how middle and senior nurse managers thought about the CiP strategy compared to how ward nurses thought about it both in terms of their awareness of and involvement in the CiP strategy. Managers, by and large, were aware of and had been involved in rolling out the strategy in programmes of work, i.e. thinking about how to boost compassion in practice. Whereas ward nurses were comparatively unaware and uninvolved in the CiP strategy, as they were busy with everyday nursing care delivery, i.e. the doing side of nursing. As the following quote from the evaluation shows, some managers were aware of this tension between thinking and doing for ward staff:

> Although most staff are aware of the Compassion in Practice, not enough is really known at floor level. The majority of the nursing staff always work to their extreme best in delivering care to patients. Lack of resources, equipment and the constant movement of having to outlie patients instead of caring for them in a safe environment often results in the interruption of the continuation of care and delays safe discharging. (Nursing middle management)

And some ward staff clearly articulated the everyday tension between doing and thinking:

> The majority of nurses have never lacked compassion but have been unable to deliver a quality of care they could be proud of due to the lack of care staff on the front line ... We do not need a strategy and more paperwork, we just need more time. (Nursing ward level)

In this book we consider the relationships at the heart of nursing: those with patients, families, co-workers and managers and the need for thinking (and practice theory) to support this approach practically. We give examples of how to balance the practical (realism) with thinking (idealism) in practice. We offer one approach to help us think afresh as nurses and nurse teachers about the relationship between thinking and doing in nursing practice, about theorising in practice: Evans et al.'s (2009) theory of recontextualisation – putting theory to work. In the following chapters, we illustrate ways in which nurses in different nursing roles think about and articulate their purpose.

Chapter overview

Chapter 2: The changing nursing workforce and the emergence of nursing knowledge

Before we discuss the conceptual underpinning of our argument in this book (Chapter 3), in Chapter 2 we introduce milestones in the history of the NHS and the national context of the NHS which have shaped nursing and nurse education. We review the changes in the nursing workforce over the last 100 years to examine how nursing knowledge has been shaped by the healthcare system. The material discussed in this chapter provides a brief overview of the social, economic and political context of our later discussion of nursing theories and how nurses theorise in practice.

This brief overview of social change and its effects on the nursing role in healthcare includes:

- Changing patterns of health and illness
- The context of nursing
- The emergence and status of modern nursing
- Education and training
- The nursing workforce

We explore how the domains of nursing, that is, our understanding of the person (client), nursing (nursing process), health, environment, care and self-care, are shaped by the social context we describe and in turn shape ways of knowing. There is some difference of opinion over the terms used to describe the broad parameters of nursing and therefore our core interest of study. We have adapted Meleis' idea of 'domain' (1991) and include caring following Leininger (1981) and self-care following Meleis (1991). Fawcett's (2005) 'essential elements' of (nursing) theory are perhaps more well-known and taught to nursing students as the metaparadigm of nursing; described by McKenna and Slevin (2008: 116) as 'the most global perspective of the discipline, a metaparadigm acting as an encapsulating framework'.

Chapter 3: Theorising in practice

In Chapter 3, we discuss learning in the workplace, and introduce the work of three theorists of knowledge who have influenced the use of nursing theory in the UK. Then we introduce theories of how knowledge develops generally before discussing two approaches which facilitate our understanding of theorising in practice which we use in the subsequent chapters:

- Ways of knowing in nursing
- 'Know-how'/'know-that'

Finally, we introduce a theoretical approach to help understand how nurses theorise in practice: Evans and Guile's theory of recontextualisation. This approach offers a way to understand how nurses may theorise in practice as they continue to contextualise and recontextualise knowledge through active learning (Evans et al., 2009, 2010).

We draw on Evans et al.'s work in Chapters 5, 6 and 7 to illustrate the ways in which nurses theorise in practice through data from a number of research studies into clinical learning, clinical practice and management.

Chapter 4: The studies

In this chapter the studies which we draw on in the following chapters to show how nurses theorise in practice are presented. There are five studies:

1. *The Leadership for Learning study* investigated how mentors and ward managers (nurse leaders) influence the ways in which student nurses learn in practice in the NHS post 2000 (Allan et al., 2007, 2011; O'Driscoll et al., 2010; Smith et al., 2010).
2. *The Delegate study* studied newly qualified nurses' learning as they transition to managing patients in acute ward areas and (importantly) managing support workers (Allan et al., 2015a, 2016a, 2018; Johnson et al., 2015; Magnusson et al., 2017).
3. *The PEGI study* investigated the professional experience of changing governance and incentive arrangements for the management of patients with long-term and complex conditions in health and social care (Allan et al., 2014; Ross et al., 2009). This study focused on interdisciplinary roles in mental health teams in the management of patients with long-term mental health conditions in the community.
4. *Developing fertility nursing roles study* explored how fertility nurses in fertility clinics practise at an extended level in specialist roles when taking on medical tasks to care holistically for infertile couples (Allan and Barber, 2004, 2005).
5. *The role of commissioning nurses or GBNs (governing body nurses) study* considered emerging new roles of senior executive nurses in clinical commissioning groups where direct nursing care is not the basis of the role (Allan et al., 2016b, 2016c, 2017; O'Driscoll et al., 2018b).

Chapters 5 and 6: Theorising in practice through workplace recontextualisation

In these chapters, we introduce activity and context which act as triggers of learning for professionals as they practise. We draw on data from the studies introduced in Chapter 4 to show how these triggers prompt learning. As presented in Chapter 3, each of the four expressions of recontextualisation (workplace, learner, pedagogy and content) sheds light on the challenges of connecting theory with practice and relating subject-based and work-based knowledge in the processes of professional learning and practice development. In Chapters 5 and 6, we focus particularly on workplace recontextualisation.

In Chapter 5, we use data from studies 1 and 2 to show how these triggers prompt learning in the workplace (clinical placement) – workplace recontextualisation. In Chapter 6, we present data from studies 3–5 on workplace recontextualisation to illustrate how experienced nurses also learn and theorise in practice and are lifelong learners.

Chapter 7: Theorising in practice through learner recontextualisation

In this chapter, we recap on learner recontextualisation. We discuss the idea of learners (at whatever stage of their career) being active partners in learning. This is key at any stage of a learner's stage of learning from school age into retirement but perhaps even more important in work-based learning programmes of professional preparation (Guile and Evans, 2010). We use data from the studies introduced in Chapter 4 to show how learners make sense of learning–learner recontextualisation.

Chapter 8: A new relationship between nursing knowledge, theory and practice

In this chapter we discuss the relationship between nursing knowledge, theories and models to explore the relationship between existing nursing knowledge, theories and practice. We don't believe such a process involves nurses *applying* theory in or to practice but developing local theories for practice. We argue (like Murphy and Smith, 2013) that such grand nursing theories should be seen as a phase of nursing theory development which helped the profession articulate its voice. We critique grand theories in nursing and revisit the relationship between nursing theory and practice. We discuss the empiricist basis of grand and mid-range theory. We discuss how our work builds on McKenna's discussion of practice theory and the development of person-centred nursing theory (Manley et al., 2011, 2014; McCormack and McCance, 2010; McCormack et al., 2008). These authors, like us, see nurses actively constructing local knowledge. Nurses, like other healthcare professionals, are lifelong, agentic learners who rework knowledge in and through local practice.

Recontextualisation theory allows us to build on previous work to illustrate how theorising takes place as learning. We discuss the findings presented in this book in the light of current educational writings on agency, identity, learning, ecologies of learning and sites of learning. We emphasise how identity as a learner and a professional are constituted through agency and context and the potential for understanding the theory–practice split as dynamic and repairable. We conclude by arguing that we need a new relationship between nursing knowledge, theory and practice.

Chapter 9: Concluding thoughts

Our purpose in writing this book has been to illustrate that nurses are lifelong learners who theorise in practice. We've argued that recontextualisation theory provides a theoretical framework for understanding nurses' theorising in practice. In this chapter we broaden our discussion of recontextualisation. We begin by discussing workplace expectations and disintegrated learning which shape workplace learning in nursing. Then we discuss how understanding learning as a *liminal* activity might deepen our understanding of learner recontextualisation and in particular, the formation and reformation of professional identity across a nurse's career.

We conclude by considering the contribution an *ecologies of learning* approach (Jackson and Barnett, 2020) might make to our understanding of workplace and learner recontextualisation.

In this concluding chapter, our intention is to start a conversation about learning in nursing from the premise that nurses theorise in practice. We argue that we need to reconceptualise the relationship between nursing knowledge, theory and practice. Throughout this chapter, we weave into our discussion what the implications of the illustrations we have given of workplace recontextualisation and learner recontextualisation in this might be for nursing.

2

The changing nursing workforce and the emergence of nursing knowledge

Chapter objectives

- Give a brief overview of social change and its effects on the nursing role in healthcare
- Explore how the changing social context shapes the domains of nursing or the fundamental concepts with which nurses understand nursing: the person (client), nursing (nursing process), health, environment, care and self-care
- Suggest ways in which the domains of nursing shape nursing knowledge

Introduction

This chapter examines how nursing knowledge and its core concepts – the person, health, environment, care and self-care – have been shaped by social changes over the last 100 years in the UK: changes in the healthcare system, in patterns of illness and disability, in people living longer, in family patterns and living arrangements, in gender roles, increased social diversity and above all, in patients' rights and expectations.

As Helen has written elsewhere, 'nursing and healthcare are essentially social activities that can be analysed from the perspective of how the individuals involved are influenced by the social world around them' (Allan et al., 2016d: 1). We discuss how these social changes have shaped the way we think about nursing in relation to the nature of the person, health, environment, care and self-care, which are acknowledged to be the focus of nursing – the core concepts on which nursing is built.

In this chapter we purposefully frame the examples of nursing knowledge and theorising which follow in the rest of this book (Chapters 5–7) within a social context to show how social constraints that exist in the workplace frame nurses' work and their efforts to make sense of theory in practice. We start by presenting a brief overview of the social changes which have shaped nursing and nurses' work in the years to 2020. We don't refer to the coronavirus pandemic in this chapter but we come back to it in our discussion in Chapters 8 and 9.

Social change and the nursing role in healthcare

Nursing in the early decades of the 21st century is remarkably similar to and, at the same time, completely different from nursing in the early 20th century: similar because it is predominantly undertaken by women and continues to involve intimate care (Smith and Allan, 2016). An example might be helping a patient to mobilise after a stroke and administering the same patient's intravenous medications. The nurse in this situation requires advanced technical skills at the same time as intimate, caring skills to enable her to interact with and care for the patient.

At the same time, nursing is completely different because nursing activities are largely not overseen or prescribed by doctors; many nurses undertake advanced skills and the nature of advanced practice has expanded exponentially to meet demands of new technologies in healthcare; nursing is less routinised and strives for an evidence base. Nurses are educated very differently too: since 2018, British nurses register as graduates although there are several other routes into nursing including the nursing associate and apprenticeship routes which offer a route to graduate registration. Also, healthcare demand is very different: people are living longer and have to manage multiple long-term conditions; survival rates over the life span have increased along with the technological potential of therapies. However, social and health inequalities, including patients' access to health services and therapies, continue to exist both within the UK and internationally (Public Health England, 2018). The Covid-19 pandemic in 2020/2021 revealed these inequalities both nationally and globally.

Perhaps the similarities and differences in nursing as it was a century ago and as it is today exist at the same time because factors such as the role of women in society, the search for an evidence base (scientific theory), technology, politics, war, the economy and the influence of medicine which shaped nursing's development as a profession have remained fairly constant over the last century:

> The discipline of nursing slowly evolved from the traditional role of women, apprenticeship, humanitarian aims, religious ideals, intuition, common sense, trial and error, theories, and research, as well as the multiple influences of medicine, technology, politics, war, economics and feminism. (Shaw, 1993: 1651)

Changing patterns of health and illness

It was first argued in the 19th century that the nature of capitalism is based on the unequal distribution of social resources and as a result, the economic base of British society, which is capitalist, exposes workers to poorer health than the wealthy in society (Allan, 2016a). This analysis is startlingly pertinent today after 10 years of austerity in the UK: health is affected by the social (including the economic) determinants of health (Dahlgren and Whitehead, 2007 [1993]; Public Health England, 2017). Reports on health inequalities have been published regularly over the last 40 years: the Black Report in 1980, the Acheson Report in 1998, the Marmot Review into Health Inequalities in 2010 and, more recently, the report of the Global Burden of Disease Study into changes in health in England between 1990 and 2013 (Newton et al., 2015), and most recently, the Marmot Review 10 Years On (2020). All of them confirm inequalities in health based on social class, ethnicity, disability, social deprivation and geography.

Other recent reports into health inequalities (Mothers and Babies: Reducing Risk through Audits and Confidential Enquiries across the UK [MBRRACE-UK], 2018; Newton et al., 2015; Public Health England, 2018) show that:

- Between 1990 and 2013, life expectancy from birth in England increased by 5.4 years from 75.9 years to 81.3 years; gains were greater for men than for women. *Gender remains a social determinant of health.*
- Rates of age-standardised years-of-life-lost (YLLs) reduced by 41.1%, whereas disability-adjusted-life-years (DALYs) were reduced by 23.8%, and years-lived-with-a-disability (YLDs) by 1.4%. *Disability remains a social determinant of health.*
- Between 1990 and 2013, the range in life expectancy in 45 regional deprivation areas remained 8.2 years for men and decreased from 7.2 years in 1990 to 6.9 years in 2013 for women. *Social deprivation remains a social determinant of health.*
- In 2005/2006, the infant mortality rate among Black groups (8.0 deaths per 1,000 live births) and Asian (6.9 deaths per 1,000 births) was significantly higher than that of white ethnic groups (Public Health England, 2018).
- Black, Asian and minority ethnic (BAME) women have significantly higher maternal and perinatal mortality rates (55% higher combined) compared to their white British counterparts (9.8%) (MBRRACE-UK, 2018). *Ethnic background remains a significant determinant of health.*

In addition, where the 19th century view of social determinants of health had been predominantly understood as structural, i.e. access to social resources determined through paid work for men, it is known that health behaviours (i.e. individuals making choices about lifestyles and behaviours acting on their own which are themselves shaped by access to resources) are a major cause of early deaths and disease into older age (Newton et al., 2015).

Although the picture of health in England in 2019 is improving, and the gap in mortality rates between men and women has reduced, the marked health inequalities between the least deprived and most deprived areas continue. Reduced mortality rates are not matched by similar reductions in morbidity, and people live longer with diseases or long-term conditions like arthritis, diabetes and heart disease. Health inequalities are avoidable; they do not occur randomly or by chance. They are socially determined by circumstances largely beyond an individual's control.

These circumstances disadvantage people and limit their chance to live longer, healthier lives. As well as policy at government level, health inequalities and changes in disease burden have implications for nurses and nursing in managing patients with long-term conditions such as asthma, diabetes, coronary heart disease, stroke, heart failure, severe mental health conditions and epilepsy.

How patients present in GP surgeries, in emergency care or outpatient departments (indeed, whether they present in the first place), shapes and constrains how nurses respond to their health needs. And nurses' responses are determined by their understanding of health, health behaviours and ethics (their knowledge and how they make sense or theorise about their work) as well as the social and interpersonal context of the nurse–patient encounter.

The context of nursing

Nursing has always been a mirror of society and constrained by the social, political and economic context including society's beliefs and structures around gender, race, ethnicity and sexual identity. Even a quick look at the photo in Figure 2.1 of nurses in training at University College Hospital, London shows how contemporary beliefs about Edwardian women shaped nursing at UCH in London at the beginning of the 20th century. Note the uniforms and the nurses' stance – how controlled, how demure and how the Sister Tutor, as the leader, is at the heart of the photo. Also, note that they are all white; they would also have been unmarried and from middle class families.

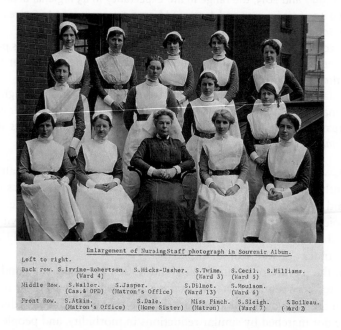

Enlargement of Nursing Staff photograph in Souvenir Album.
Left to right.
Back row. S.Irvine-Robertson. S.Hicks-Ussher. S.Twine. S.Cecil. S.Williams.
         (Ward 4)   (Ward 3) (Ward 5)
Middle Row. S.Waller.   S.Jasper.   S.Dilnot.   S.Moulson.
         (Cas.& OPD) (Matron's Office) (Ward 13) (Ward 6)
Front Row. S.Atkin.   S.Dale.   Miss Finch. S.Sleigh.   S.Boileau.
         (Matron's Office) (Home Sister) (Matron)   (Ward 7)   (Ward 2)

Figure 2.1   Nurses in training at University Hospital London, early 20th century

Reproduced with kind permission of the 'UCH London Nurses' Charity 2019

The NHS remains heavily gendered with 41% men and 59% women employed; in nursing, men make up 10–11% of total registered nurses and have done for over a century. Those male nurses who are registered (and they are still called male nurses as if to signify that they are different, unusual) are over-represented in specialities such as mental health and acute care and in higher earning management positions – seemingly because these are more gender-appropriate roles for male nurses (Wilkinson and Miers, 1999). A recent NHS Improvement report (2019) on the NHS gender pay gap showed that women in the NHS on average earn 23% less than men:

- An average full-time female worker is paid £28,702 a year in basic salary compared to £37,470 average pay for men – a gap of more than 23%.
- Male doctors can expect to be paid £67,788 in basic pay compared to £57,569 for female doctors.
- 6.5 times as many male medical consultants as female received the top platinum bonus worth £77,000 a year.

Similar trends are present for BAME staff employed in the NHS across medicine, nursing, midwifery and allied health professions:

- Diversity across the NHS is above the national average, with BAME staff making up 17% of the non-medical NHS workforce. However, only 11% of senior managers are BAME. This drops to 6.4% at a very senior level (NHS, 2018).

In addition to gender and ethnicity, health and social policy are hugely important in shaping the context in which nurses work. More recently, the global economic crisis has seen governments adopting increasingly 'managerialist' agendas (Rudge, 2015). These agendas entrenched dominant forms of health delivery – namely biomedicine – as well as cut funding for healthcare provision. The resulting budget cuts are couched in the language of efficiency savings and the effective use of resources. Alongside these financial constraints and changes in funding of services, governments in Western Europe have also been concerned with transforming the control of public services (Davies et al., 2005; Smith et al., 2012) and restructuring the relationships within traditional systems of governance (Saltman, 2003). Within this context, the concept of a commissioning board as a governance model for healthcare has emerged in many European systems (Saltman and Figueras, 1997). This managerialist agenda has been introduced by governments of all political persuasions.

In the UK, the Health and Social Care Act (Department of Health [DH], 2012) introduced a major restructuring of the NHS in England. This included removing responsibility from government ministers for direct operational management and creating Clinical Commissioning Groups (CCGs) to plan, agree and monitor health services. In 2013, led primarily by general practitioners (GPs), CCGs took over the design and commissioning of most health services in England on the assumption that commissioning by clinicians would lead to improved decision-making, improved outcomes for patients and more effective use of resources (DH, 2011). CCGs have a legal duty to assure quality across commissioned services in secondary care and, from 2015/2016, have additional optional responsibilities including general practice performance management and reviewing GP contracts (Holder et al., 2015). These arrangements changed again in 2019 as GP practices became reorganised into primary care networks as part of the renegotiations of the GP contract by the Conservative government under Prime Minister Theresa May.

A concomitant change which has occurred with increased marketisation and managerialist control of the NHS has been the change in patient agency in health-care. In the 1990s, following the Patient's Charter (DH, 1995) and the Expert Patients Programme (DH, 2001), nursing positioned itself as the voice and advocate of the patient. More recently, this inadvisable and frankly naïve position has been abandoned and more robust systems have been introduced to enable patients and carers to speak out for themselves (DH, 2000). The patient is both expected to be and expects to be more active in their care; although of course this varies depending on the social and cultural capital that patients have access to (May et al., 2014).

The inherent contradiction in the rise of greater patient choice and the expecta-tion of patient agency within the context of managerialism since 2008 has actually placed nurses under intense pressure (Jones and Kelly, 2014; Paley, 2014; Smith, 2013). The situation has been made worse by reports from several inquiries into:

- disastrous patient outcomes due to poor nursing and medical care (Francis, 2013)
- appalling oversight and governance from hospital trust management and a culture of intimidation and bullying (Harding Clark, 2006; Hazell, 2015; Jackson et al., 2012).

We will now consider the emergence of nursing and its current status in the UK which has shaped how nurses think, what knowledge they draw on and how they theorise and therefore (We argue) what they see as their professional discipline and therefore their responsibility.

The emergence and status of modern nursing

One of the meanings of to nurse was to care for the infirm and was associated primar-ily with women as caring skills were those ascribed to women in traditional cultures, i.e. bathing, cooking, intimate care of bodies, feeding, growing herbs (Oakley, 1986). Cross-culturally, another group of women who nursed were religious women who dedicated themselves to service as part of a religious function outside the family. Men also nursed when women were not available, as part of their military functions or in spaces where women were banned (in monasteries or in prisons).

Christianity and Islam produced dedicated nurses before the foundation of modern nursing. Modern, secular nursing emerged in the 19th century in the UK and Germany, spreading rapidly to the rest of Europe and the United States. Modern, professional (that is, non-religious, employed or paid) nurses across Western Europe, the UK and the USA remained for the large part, white, middle class women (as the picture in Figure 2.1 shows) with recruits into nursing support roles for working class, Black and ethnic minority women (Wilkinson and Miers, 1999). Modern nursing struggled, and still struggles, with its image as predominantly female, its association with care of the body which is deeply stigmatised in many cultures (Allan, 2016b) and its image as the helpmate to medical men (Ehrenreich and English, 1979; Franklin, 2014). These stereotypical images of nursing are remarkably persistent (ten Hoeve et al., 2013). In a presentation in 2021 by Professor Michael Traynor on some research undertaken in 2012, he recounted how a senior nurse at NHS England explained nursing's lack of professional status: 'Nursing is the only profession where being seen as intelligent is seen as a hindrance' (Personal communication).

There is disagreement amongst nurses about how to challenge these stereotypes. Between educationalists and research active nurses, there are those who feel nurses are professionals in the same sense as medicine and aspire to professional status, argue for higher levels of education, research-based practice and restricted entry to nurse education programmes. Among practitioners and managers, there are those who seek to unite all those employed in nursing and caring work as a unionised occupational grouping; nurse managers who seek to embed nursing management within a dominant managerialist discourse; and practitioners who justify nurses' roles in modern healthcare through advanced practice. Unfortunately, this has led to a lack of a coherent body of disciplinary knowledge in nursing, which has been a major stumbling block (ironically) to nursing being viewed as a profession and latterly, nursing's entry to university as a discipline. It was against this background that early nurse theorists wrote their grand theories of nursing and nursing models.

In addition, the need for an expanding nursing workforce has led to a large and growing migrant workforce across the West and in developing wealthier countries. This migration has further entrenched existing discriminatory patterns of behaviour in nursing based on social class and increased racism and discrimination cross-culturally (Allan and Westwood, 2015; Grant and Guerin, 2018; Walani, 2015). There are tensions between nursing support workers and registered nurses who now work in complex nursing teams where boundaries between doctors/nurses and between nurses/ nursing support workers have become increasingly blurred (Magnusson et al., 2017).

Lastly in this section on the emergence and status of nursing, the status of nursing in the UK suffered an enormous blow at the time of the Francis Report into poor care at Mid Staffordshire Hospitals (Francis, 2013) and the report of the investigations into the of abuse of learning disabled residents at the Winterbourne View Hospital (NHS England, 2014). Pervasive deficiencies were identified in the provision of compassionate care (Francis, 2013). The effects of the Francis Report were still being felt by front-line nurses in 2018 when Helen and colleagues evaluated the *Compassion in Practice Vision and Strategy* (DH, 2013) on nursing, midwifery and care staff. This initiative was itself a reaction by the Chief Nurse for England to head off criticisms of nurses. A data extract which illustrates this blow to nurses' self-confidence follows:

> I found it incredibly, it was soul destroying when I read the Francis report. (Ward manager acute care NHS Hospital Trust)

Education and training

One of the recommendations of the Francis Report was to change the culture in hospitals by promoting and demanding a patient safety culture from all staff based on a number of shared values, including compassion. Francis reported a failure to provide fundamental care by nurses and nursing support staff; nurse education programmes were criticised for not providing sufficient time in professional preparation programmes for students to become proficient in practical patient care. Another criticism of the professional preparation of nurses was the (supposed) failure to recruit only those able to demonstrate compassion. The criticism of nurse education prompted the *Shape of Caring: A Review of the Future Education and Training of Registered Nurses and Care* (Health Education England [HEE]/Nursing and Midwifery Council [NMC], 2015). This report largely exonerated nursing professional preparation curricula. However the NMC (2013) disagreed and in their report post Francis, stated:

> We fully support the recommendation that there should be an increased focus in nurse training, education and professional development on the practical requirements of delivering compassionate care in addition to the theory. (NMC, 2013: 14)

Essentially, the NMC upheld Francis's criticism of nurse education; their 2013 report stated that nursing education had to change because insufficient attention had been paid in nursing curricula to the practicalities of nursing. As a result, student nurses and midwives recruited to professional preparation programmes are expected to have the capacity to deliver high quality compassionate care (DH, 2013). This involved a change from previous selection to programmes where students were initially shortlisted according to their intellectual ability measured by previous academic success – not unreasonably given that all nurse education moved into universities in the mid-1990s and since 2012 in the UK, all nurses qualify as a registered nurse with a Bachelor degree. Since the Francis Report and the NMC's Response, a clear emphasis is now placed on selecting nurses and midwives for training based on caring values, including compassion and empathy, as well as technical and academic skills (DH, 2013). This recruitment strategy was launched under the name values-based recruitment, or VBR, as if to differentiate post Francis from pre Francis nurse recruitment. Values have always been used by admissions tutors in nursing and other healthcare professional preparation programmes. Imagine the values used by the admissions sister tutor in the photo above! However the language used to describe VBR implied that the correct values had not been used in the past.

We argued earlier that there have always been different groups in nursing who argue over nursing's purpose; the different responses by stakeholders like the NMC and the Willis Commission to the Francis Report show these different groups in play. In some respects, the response to the Francis Report is an echo of the arguments put forward at the introduction of Project 2000 and replayed on the move of nursing into universities (Smith and Allan, 2010). There have existed since the start of modern professional nursing (at least in the UK) differences in opinion about what the 'best' training might be; Florence Nightingale had very different views to Mrs Bedford-Fenwick in the early 20th century. This has continued through the introduction of Project 2000 (following the Judge Report in 1985 [RCN, 1985a, 1985b]) in the early 1990s. It was intended that the P2K nurse would be educated to become the knowledgeable doer who would be able to respond to a changing healthcare environment. Fairly rapidly, following sustained but unsubstantiated criticism of P2K students and newly qualified nurses, the Fitness for Practice (F4P) curriculum was introduced in the late 1990s to address the perceived imperfections of the P2K nurse and curriculum. The F4P curriculum scaled back the academic aspirations of P2K and reinstated a practice focus on skills. And latterly, after the move into higher education, there has been sustained and continued criticism of the location of nursing education in universities supported to some extent by the NMC standards for education in nursing and midwifery in 2009 and 2018.

One final piece of the background to nurse education is important for the argument in this book. That is the short lasting introduction of supernumerary status under P2K which was intended to release all students from an apprenticeship model of learning. This had a hugely detrimental effect on nurse staffing in the NHS as nursing assistants (unregulated and frequently unsupervised support workers) were employed to replace student nurses on clinical rotas. It gave rise to some of the conflict described above between unregistered and registered staff whose conditions of work and opportunities for career development and promotion were very different. This leads us into the final section on the changing nursing workforce.

Changing nursing workforce

Nursing has always adapted to the demands of patients, the medical profession and managers. As Sandelowski (2000) has argued, 'new' roles are not new; nurses have always taken on new technologies as they emerge to adapt to change. In the process, they learn new skills, discard old ones and in many cases, integrate new with old skills. A report by Read et al. (2001) into new roles in practice (the ENRIP study) suggested that in 1997 (the year of the survey) there were an estimated 3,000 new nursing roles in practice. The criterion for inclusion was the presence of a degree of innovation in the new role as assessed by Heads of Nursing in participating NHS trusts.

This process of adaptation has had to speed up as the clinical workplace becomes increasingly technologised. This is recognised in NHS England's plan to develop a healthcare workforce that is proficient, knowledgeable and possesses advanced clinical skills which can contribute to multidisciplinary working (Kaur et al., 2016). While technology was part and parcel of nursing in Nightingale's time, e.g. the devolving of temperature taking to nurses from doctors, the rate at which new technologies are introduced has increased exponentially. With ongoing challenges in retaining junior doctors and increasingly complex needs of patients worldwide, there is a drive to develop and upskill nurses to occupy advanced clinical roles (Gray, 2016). More recently, in response to a public inquiry of inadequate quality care (Roberts, 2013) and the need for effective leadership to influence and inspire change in healthcare delivery (Muls et al., 2015), it is expected by NHS England that Advanced Nurse Practice (ACP) roles may be a catalyst for healthcare service improvement as they aspire to provide individualised, safe and effective care for patients with complex needs (Imison et al., 2016; Maclaine, 2017). All of this has framed the professional preparation of nurses (and other healthcare workers) as well as the curricula and knowledge base for practice.

Even in this relatively short discussion of the emergence of nursing as a profession, it can be seen that nursing has been through tumultuous change over the last century, as outlined briefly above. These changes have had an effect on:

- how nurses think about the agency and experience of being a patient and how this shapes our thinking and practice around care and self-care
- how we think about the nature of personhood and autonomy, decision-making for health and responsibility for health outcomes
- thinking about health and the effects of the environment on health in the context of climate crisis.

The nature of the person, health, environment, care and self-care: fundamental building blocks of nursing theory

Nursing models and theories were developed and introduced to nursing curricula in Western Europe, Australia, Japan, Canada and America in the 20th century. At the heart of all nursing theories are some fundamental concepts about the nature of nursing or the metaparadigm of nursing (Fawcett, 1992; Fitzpatrick and Whall, 1996). The metaparadigm of any discipline (and nursing therefore) is 'the most global perspective of the discipline acting as an encapsulating ... framework' (McKenna and Slevin, 2008: 116). Fawcett's (2005) 'essential elements' of (nursing) theory which she argues form the metaparadigm of nursing are well-known; it includes four key 'elements' or concepts: *person, health, nursing, environment*. There is some difference of opinion over the domains of nursing and therefore our core interest of study because the nature of nursing has changed over time as shown in this chapter. Thus changes in patterns of health and illness and social changes have meant the definition of nursing has changed over time and so have these elements (Meleis, 1992; Murphy and Smith, 2013: Vol. 3). We therefore include *person, health, environment, nursing* and *care* and *self-care* in our discussion of the elements which form the domains of nursing. And we retain *environment* and widen this to include climate crisis.

In 1966, Henderson's definition stated that:

> The unique function of the nurse is to assist the individual, sick or well, in the performance of those activities contributing to health or its recovery (or to peaceful death) that he [*sic*] would perform unaided if he had the necessary strength, will or knowledge. (Henderson, 1966: 15)

Forty-six years later, the International Council of Nurses' (ICN) definition in 2002 stated that:

> Nursing encompasses autonomous and collaborative care of individuals of all ages, families, groups and communities, sick or well and in all settings. Nursing includes the

promotion of health, prevention of illness, and the care of ill, disabled and dying people. Advocacy, promotion of a safe environment, research, participation in shaping health policy and in patient and health systems management, and education are also key nursing roles.

Note how the definition and thus the expected role of nursing has changed: a move from unique function to collaborative care; the inclusion of disability in the ICN definition; a move from assisting activities of daily living to autonomous care across all settings. The language of the 2002 definition is also more inclusive of gender, families and communities. The focus in the ICN definition is on a far broader field of practice including health promotion, health prevention and health policy rather than focused on the individual. Many nursing roles have shifted from the everyday delivery of care to the delivery and supervision of care in increasingly complex teams. However even with these changes in nurses' roles, the ICN's definition still encompasses care as a fundamental element of nursing. Caring (about) and care/ing (for) remain significant elements of nursing's ideals, values and underpinning philosophy (NMC, 2018b). '[F]ew could argue that care is not an integral part of the nature of nursing' (Bassett, 2004: 17). As we will see, even where nurses focus on commissioning healthcare, they still care about and care for patients (albeit at the population level) in their collaborative decisions about healthcare. Writing this during winter 2020, perhaps this strategic and policy level caring is particularly in our minds at this moment of the Covid pandemic when global and policy action in nursing are integral to population health.

So, we suggest the fundamental concepts which shape the nature of nursing may be said to be:

- The *person* – the patient is now considered to have agency and to be responsible for maintaining his/her own health and wellbeing. However, the degree to which patients are understood to be agentic persons once they become ill or disabled is open to interpretation.
- *Health* encompasses a holistic view of health including an individual's health, family and community health where appropriate and health promotion in a wider societal sense.
- The *environment* (including the climate crisis) and the relationship between the person, families and communities in their environment.
- *Nursing* is a service based on an interpersonal process between person and nurse where the goal is for the person (patient) to feel cared for and for the nurse to feel supported to care.
- *Care* – nursing care is delivered in a thoughtful and systematic way – the model for delivery of care is often the nursing process.
- *Self-care* – the person being cared for works with nurses to shape and co-produce person-centred care. This is perhaps the most recent concept largely because the person was considered for many years to inhabit a patient role where enforced passivity was expected.

The integration of these domains into nursing curricula and practice in the UK as the basis of theory has been a struggle (McKenna, 1997; Murphy and Smith, 2013: Vol. 2) despite views to the contrary (Bradshaw and Merriman, 2008). We think this is partly because the domains of nursing as they are set out in nursing theorists' work are not what the UK's regulatory body for nursing, the Nursing and Midwifery Council (NMC), means when it refers to domains. The NMC talks of values, skill clusters and domains as competences rather than building blocks of theory. This has been made even more difficult since the Francis Report (see above) where the lack of dignified care delivery was (partly) blamed on the failure of nurse education to equip student nurses with practical competencies to meet standards of skills and competence. In reaction to this and building on the NMC's existing focus on skills and competencies, a renewed emphasis was placed on a component of care, compassion, and incorporated into the NMC Standards (NMC, 2018a) and competencies. These competencies are thought to (somehow) encourage compassion and are emphasised at the expense of the domains of nursing underpinning nursing theories. The domains of *nursing*, as far as it informs the delivery of care, i.e. the nursing process, and *health* were perhaps most fully integrated into curricula and practice. Although, in practical terms, they are more frequently an aspiration rather than part of the living curriculum. Where the domains were influential was in the shaping and articulation of *nursing knowledge for practice* in the UK in the development of practice development in the 1990s and person-centred theory in the 2000s.

Conclusion

In this chapter we've discussed how nursing knowledge and its core concepts – the person, health, environment, care and self-care – have been shaped by social changes over the last 100 years in the UK. In doing so, we have set up the following chapters where nurses' thinking (and theorising in practice) is examined in different workplace settings. We argue that while the workplace context may change, nurses' theorising may not. We give working examples to illustrate how nurses theorise across different workplaces at different stages of their careers.

In McKenna's book on nursing theory (1997), he aimed to critically evaluate nursing theory through exploring how theory 'should' take place. He argued that practice theory, or theorising in practice, has been ignored in favour of 'off the shelf' theories. He advocates person-centred theory for nursing based on nurses' ability to theorise and the practice of theorising in practice. Our argument in this book builds on McKenna's argument for practice theorising and person-centred care theory (Manley et al., 2011; McCormack and McCance, 2010; McCormack et al., 2008). We argue that Evans et al.'s (2009) theory of recontextualisation offers a way to understand how nurses learn and thus how they theorise, and practice theory develops.

In Chapter 3 we introduce theories of knowledge and describe Evans and Guile's ideas of knowledge recontextualisation to develop our understanding of local practice knowledge for nursing practice. We will show how knowledge making and theorising take place in practice in different settings in emerging roles within complex teams. However (following McKenna, 1997), given the pressures on nurses in the healthcare system today, we acknowledge that many nurses are surviving not theorising – that is, they are not routinely offered opportunities to theorise and share observations on theory and knowledge in practice. The research interviews we draw on to illustrate their theorising were elicited during breaks from routine, but they show (a) that nurses theorise if offered the opportunity, and (b) the potential for developing practice theory which is remarkably person-centred (despite all the constraints on their time). Perhaps this is because as Manley et al. (2014) argue, relationships are at the heart of person-centred care: those with patients, families, co-workers and managers. Manley et al.'s (2014) notion of 'shared purpose' in practice development is one way to show how thinking critically guides nursing action in person-centred care. Our ideas in this book build on Manley's work in developing ideas around knowledge by drawing on theories of knowledge recontextualisation.

3

Theorising in practice

Chapter objectives

- Discuss learning in the workplace
- Introduce the work of three theorists of knowledge who have influenced the use of nursing theory in the UK (Lev Vygotsky, 1896–1934; John Dewey, 1859–1952; Michael Eraut, 1940–2018)
- Introduce theories of how knowledge develops
- Discuss the concepts of knowledge and ways of knowing which are fundamental to our understanding of theorising in practice
- Present Evans et al.'s (2009) theory of recontextualisation (see also Evans, 2015; Evans and Guile, 2012) used to facilitate our understanding of theorising in practice

Introduction

We believe that the social context informs how nurses think and talk about theory and perhaps just as importantly, how nurses theorise. Thus a brief overview of the social context of nursing was presented in Chapter 2. We also discussed how the social context shapes the domains of nursing and the educational theories which inform nursing theory in the UK. In this chapter, we introduce some thoughts about knowledge before setting out the theoretical framework used in this book to inform the following chapters where we illustrate how nurses theorise in practice. We start by a brief overview of learning in the workplace.

Learning in the workplace

In order for full engagement in learning to occur for the student, workplace learning needs to be fully situated in three ways:

1. in practical activity
2. in the culture and context of the workplace learning environment
3. in the socio-biographical features of the learner's life (Evans et al., 2006).

Other features of learning critical to full engagement in the workplace learning environment include engagement from mentors or supervisors or those responsible for learning; as well as engagement in the workplace generally so that all workers are supportive of learning (Spouse, 1998). Nursing in the UK, as we have seen in Chapter 2, has a particular social context which has shaped learning for nursing students. Relationships between nursing students and registered staff were traditionally hierarchical with the apprentice low down the hierarchy and not seen or treated as core members of the ward team. Unfortunately, the introduction of supernumerary status in the late 1990s has not led to greater inclusion in ward teams or more engaged learning or supervisory relationships (Allan et al., 2011). Student nurses are now seen primarily as students, they are not seen as workers who might be included in ward teams in all clinical placements. Innovations such as communities of practice were an attempt to modernise relationships between learner and supervisor/mentor (Spouse, 1998, 2001a, 2001b). But the success of such innovations has been variable exactly because students are not seen as part of the workforce (Evans and Kelly, 2004). Many of these contextual features of the British workplace learning for student nurses is replicated internationally (James and Chapman, Dec 2009/Jan 2010).

Solomon et al. (2006) argue that the term 'workplace learning' has particular kinds of meanings and practices because of its location external to an educational institution where learning may not be the primary focus in workplaces. It cannot be assumed that learning in the workplace will take place without structure and support (Scheeres et al., 2010). Or that learners will necessarily be signposted to learning or be able to identify learning opportunities. Melia (2006) argued that, while nurse educators often assume that the NHS is a learning organisation, in fact, the NHS is primarily focused on patient care or, in these neoliberal times, patient throughput (Davies et al., 2005; Rudge, 2015). Perhaps as importantly, while the NHS may not be formally focused on learning, neither does it attend sufficiently to the informal learning which occurs in the workplace for learners. Nursing students learn poor practice from informal learning opportunities as well as good practice (Groothuizen et al., 2019). The lack of awareness and acknowledgement of the importance of informal learning and its potential as an untapped source of learning in the workplace is also recognised outside nursing (Bockarie, 2002).

As a result of this neglect of learning in the NHS, we would adapt Chisholm's general observation about workplace learning (2008:142) to say that:

> Our understandings of what is to be learned [in the NHS] do not take much account of who is learning and for what purposes – so we do not have much of a rational basis for working out how and where learning, for what and for whom, might best take place [in the NHS].

To address this lack of knowledge about learning in the workplace, Chisholm (2008: 142) suggests a 'positive borderlessness' which might help learning within practice disciplines to:

> Re-focus and reposition the conceptual and practical connections between learning subjects (who), learning sites (where) and learning pathways (when and how). In contrast to the negative connotations of 'Entgrenzung' (de-bordering), positive borderlessness situates learning as more extensive (lifelong), more specialised (life-near), more differentiated (lifewide), more flexible, more individualised and more contingent.

An example of de-bordering is the implicit belief in the NHS and nurse education that professional preparation programmes prepare students for registration and to work as a registered nurse immediately upon registration. The phrase used frequently is 'to hit the ground running'. This is based on an assumption that the learning needs to reach a point at which it is complete so that a registrant is safe and can be certified as safe to practise. We challenge this assumption in this book to show that professional learning continues and should continue throughout a career for safe practice even if interrupted by life events (Evans et al., 2004).

A distinguishing feature of workplace learning in the NHS is (a) the busy and emotional nature of the work with the consequent lack of time to debrief either about the emotions which may shape that experience or any possible learning, and (b) the lack of learning experiences in workplaces with a high number of students to accommodate in busy wards and clinics with overstretched staff and a lack of supervision. The busyness, the lack of staff to foster learning and the pressure on work placements can lead to poor horizontal and vertical learning where students struggle to put knowledge to work through a lack of opportunity (Groothuizen et al., 2019).

One final thought about learning in the workplace. Current models in many professions fail to address knowledge (Quinlan and Song, 1998). Quinlan and Song argue that current models of learning in the workplace are largely a method for the development of competences or motor skills as we show in this book. Such models do not focus on the knowledge base required for practice or how a student and new professional becomes a member of a community of practice. Our theoretical framework, the theory of recontextualisation or putting knowledge to work (Evans et al., 2009), focuses on the development of adult vocational learners through exploring the linkages between learning and knowledge production as well as the development of competence and the student's role in the learning process.

Knowledge for practice

We argue that while knowledge remains central to nursing practice and teaching, nursing cannot and does not limit itself to nursing knowledge but draws on other disciplinary knowledge to create localised, practice nursing knowledge. This does not mean that nurses will reject post-positivist knowledge or formal theories; that would make no sense. There are facts which can be applied to a range of contexts and settings but they should be viewed critically as part of multiple ways of knowing (Porter, 1995, 1998; Purkis and Bjornsdottir, 2006). Many earlier nursing theories were dominated by rationalist and empirical worldviews, the 'upshot [of which] was that the knowledge being developed [in nursing] was fragmented and un-unified' (Kikuchi and Simmons, 1992: 2, cited by McKenna 1997: 45). The limitations of evidence-based approaches to nursing which are based on a post-positivist view of the science are an example of rationalism and emiricism which fails to fully illuminate nursing in all its richness. Evidence-based theories are not infrequently founded on theories of pathophysiology but are applied to the nursing context by nurses as they theorise in practice. In Box 3.1, an example of the tension in applying post-positivist knowledge in nursing is shown.

Box 3.1   Theorising in practice

Consider the following scenario where medical and nursing clinicians in intensive care struggle with their empirical knowledge (disturbing a patient results in reduced blood pressure) and ethical and aesthetic knowing (the patient needs a wash, moving and making comfortable):

A patient is critically ill and supported by inotropic support to maintain his blood pressure. He's ventilated and sedated. On the ward round that morning, the physicians and nursing team discuss whether to disturb him for nursing care. The physician argues not to 'as his BP drops whenever we touch him'. The nurse looking after the patient argues to carry on and deliver nursing care as he feels the patient should be washed and cared for.

This example is drawn from Helen's experience as an intensive care nurse where she recognised the importance of facts but equally of context when tacit and ethical knowing come into tension with evidence-based medicine or rationalist/empiricist knowledge.

Practice knowledge, produced and reproduced through practice knowing in local settings for local purposes by individual and groups of nurses making sense of new roles, challenges the 'old' ideas of what nurses should be doing when they nurse. But it also challenges accepted views of what forms of knowledge are valued (Purkis and Bjornsdottir, 2006). To enable nurses to produce and value nursing knowledge which emerges in practice, we need to educate nurses to be active learners and co-producers of knowledge for practice. Practice might then be informed legitimately by theory as nurses contextualise and recontextualise or rework knowledge in new settings with each and every patient. Later in this chapter, we introduce a theoretical approach to knowledge for practice, Evans et al.'s theory of knowledge recontextualisation, to develop our understanding of local practice knowledge for nursing practice. Before that, three theories of learning which have influenced nursing theory and curricula in the UK are briefly discussed.

Theorists of learning

Important theorists of knowledge and learning who have been influential in writings on nursing knowledge include Lev Vygotsky, John Dewey and Michael Eraut. Dewey had an influence on earlier American nursing theorists whereas Vygotsky and Eraut have been more influential on writing on nurse education in the UK from the 1970s onwards.

Vygotsky was a Russian psychologist who developed a theory of socio-cultural or active learning (Vygotsky and Luria, 1930). Two key features of his work have been important in nursing: situated learning and the relationship between learner and supervisor or mentor (Sanders and Welk, 2005; Spouse, 1998). He was interested in the socio-cultural context in which learning takes place, which he called situated learning; and importantly, in the interactions within what he called the 'zone of proximal development' which was key to learning in children. His work was developed with children but has been applied to nursing education (Spouse, 1998; Thomas, 2013) in ways that explore and develop how informal learning takes place when 'students abandon formalised knowledge in order to deal with the messiness of the situation at hand and rely upon informal or tacit understandings and coaching from an expert' (Spouse, 1998: 260). As Spouse argues, Vygotsky's theory illuminates informal learning in nursing practice and the role of the mentor in clinical practice. It should perhaps be said that the application of Vygotsky's work in nursing has been rather uncritical as, ironically, while his work argues for greater understanding of the social context in which children learn, the rather constrained context in which student nurses learn is somewhat glossed over in much of this applied work.

The works of Vygotsky are linked to social constructivism, which, according to Abdal-Haqq (1999), offers a theoretical perspective on learning and meaning-making, not teaching, with an explanation of the nature of knowledge and how humans learn in social and cultural contexts. A fundamental principle of constructivism is that what we learn is associated with the interpretation of our experiences in relation to new information and how it connects to old information. Learning occurs as individuals construct their own new understandings or knowledge through interaction with and reflection on what they already know and believe, balanced against the ideas, events, people and activities they have contact with in their day-to-day activities. As Abdal-Haqq notes, constructivist approaches are regarded as producing greater internalisation and deeper understanding than traditional teaching methods.

John Dewey (1933) was an American philosopher who argued that knowledge should be applied to everyday life in a practical way through lived experience

(Gramling, 2004; LeVasseur, 1999). He was a pragmatist who believed that theory could or should be seen to work in practice and, therefore, be adaptive.

Dewey's ideas were influential as they coincided with an explosion of interest in experiential clinical knowledge within the nursing academy (Fairman, 2008). Fairman (1997) cites Virginia Henderson as an example in this tradition of drawing on practical knowledge to develop theory. More recent work by Rolfe (2014) emphasises the importance of Dewey's insights into reflection for nursing:

> For Dewey, reflection is not simply having an experience and then going home to think about it. On the contrary, thinking is an active process that involves forming hypotheses and trying them out here and now in the real world. Thinking or reflection is therefore a form of experimentation. We cannot reflect in an armchair; reflection can only take place in practice; reflection, in Dewey's words, involves: doing something overtly to bring about the anticipated result, and thereby testing the hypothesis. (Dewey, 1916: 115 cited by Rolfe, 2014: 1179–1180)

For Rolfe, there has been both an overemphasis in nursing on reflection but also an incorrect use of reflection. He argues that reflection in nursing is skewed towards reflection-on-action, i.e. after the event, and is never experimental or fully emancipatory. Thus knowledge is not generated in practice or, at least, not encouraged or articulated. Our data show that it is indeed experimental and emancipatory across a wide range of settings.

Early nurse theorist Hildegarde Peplau was influenced by Dewey's work and his focus on relationships. However, she believed his understanding of *learning as doing* was too restrictive – it failed in her eyes to incorporate feeling, which is integral to learning. From this insight, she developed her understanding of learning as an outcome of the development of the nurse–patient relationship (Fairman, 2008), i.e. learning as feeling and doing. An overemphasis on thinking as doing has led to the recurring seesawing between skills and thinking curricula in nursing – recently articulated in the resistance to acquiring skills in simulated labs rather than with patients, when we know that simulations are good for learning in nursing (Forber et al., 2015).

The third theorist is Michael Eraut (1994), who identified knowledge in practice as three interacting and closely connected forms of knowledge:

1. Process knowledge (skilled behaviour and deliberation)
2. Personal knowledge (impressions and experiential interpretations)
3. Propositional knowledge (theories, concepts and propositions)

These different strands or forms of knowledge together create professional knowledge. Work on knowledge and knowledge transfer influenced the development of practice theories (Manley and Webster, 2006). Eraut's writing on tacit knowing was particularly influential (Eraut, 2000) in this tradition as it recognised, validated and integrated practice knowledge (Rutter, 2009). Eraut's work on knowledge transfer across cultures was also important in the 1990s in nurse education as more focus was given to students' learning across different clinical areas and between academic sites of learning and practice (Eraut, 1994; Eraut et al., 1995, 1996). His ideas around knowledge transfer became increasingly important as the place of learning changed when nursing moved from nursing colleges attached to hospitals to university departments. He argued that the integration of knowledge learnt at university into workplaces depended on the ways in which different forms of knowledge were valued by each setting. During this period of curricular change where the locus of learning moved from nursing colleges attached to hospitals to universities (see Chapter 2), his work on knowledge transfer across cultures was helpful. His work suggested a way of understanding the 'split' between nurse education and nursing practice.

Before knowledge and ways of knowing are considered, we briefly explore how knowledge develops.

How knowledge develops

Our view of how knowledge develops is historicist, that is we understand knowledge to be shaped by social context which changes over time. Knowledge isn't received uncritically but shaped by key influencing agents and interests. Firstly, all knowledge (in this case, nursing knowledge for practice and teaching) is contextual, shaped by contextual knowing (situated learning). Helen particularly has been influenced here by psychodynamic understandings of how we learn as human beings who are shaped by emotions in the learning process (Jacobs, 1991). This psychodynamic turn is also influenced by critical theory and critical reflection with its concern with emancipatory knowledge (Avis and Freshwater, 2006; Freshwater and Rolfe, 2001) and by the potential of psychodynamic supervision for learning (Allan, 2011). In Helen's experience, knowledge may be emancipatory: that is, knowledge gained through practice, teaching or research can illuminate dominant forms of knowledge which privilege those groups in society who are more powerful and give voice to those who are oppressed.

Two examples of emancipatory nursing research which illustrate oppressive power structures within nursing and healthcare are:

- Annette Street's (1992) ethnography of operating department nursing, *Inside Nursing*, where she illuminates nurses' voices in this area of practice which is dominated by surgeons and rife with oppressive practices between surgeons and nurses and between nurses themselves.
- Jocelyn Lawler's (1991) book *Behind the Screens*, where she explores the nursing of the body and how this work has been hidden and why.

In our view, emancipatory knowledge arises both from reflection-in-action and reflection-on-action if thinking and doing are grounded *in practice*. It grows from reflection to construction of new knowledge – theorising in practice. We have argued elsewhere that we don't find the contribution of Benner and Tanner (1987) sufficient as it suggests that nurses think reflectively but act on intuitive knowledge (Allan et al., 2018). The purpose of this book is to show that nurses articulate this intuitive knowledge in theorising in practice at the same time as thinking while doing – reflecting. Whether they are given time to articulate this thinking and reflection and, thus, to theorise routinely in and on practice/action is another question.

So for us, knowledge development is a dynamic social activity (even where pursued on one's own) and there are no objective truths which are final or permanent. This interpretative-constructionist approach to knowledge development informed by a critical view of knowledge development means that while we accept the rationalist and empiricist worldviews as far as they offer ways to understand knowledge, in evidence-based nursing for example, they are too restrictive in their understanding of what counts as knowledge. An empiricist, even a post-positivist view of the world, does not (in our view) account for the complexities of, and dynamics in, nursing. As Meleis (1991) argues, knowledge doesn't progress in evolutionary or revolutionary ways but is convolutionary – it has its ups and downs, twists and turns and doesn't develop in a linear progress. There are multiple strands which are context specific and, at the same time, universally transferrable. For further exploration of these views of knowledge development see Murphy and Smith (2013: Vols 1–3).

Ways of knowing

As a nurse, Helen has always been interested in how knowledge is used and/or applied in practice. Reading sociology for her undergraduate degree, Helen was interested in how knowledge was acted upon, not in theory as an end in itself necessarily. So even when reading grand theory (e.g. Marxist theory) with its orientation to philosophy and theory of social change (revolution), she asked herself, how might this theory be used in everyday nursing? Helen was introduced to thinking about knowledge while studying for her Diploma in Nursing at the Royal College of Nursing in the 1980s as an intensive care ward sister. A key reading for her Diploma was Carper's 'Fundamental patterns of knowing' (1978), which sets out the different types of knowing in nursing.

Reading Carper's paper was the first time Helen felt she was aware of the difference in knowing (where her feelings about what she was experiencing in relation to patients' conditions and nursing were described) and knowledge (where the empirical medical knowledge she had learned on her post-registration ICU course unfolded in front of her eyes) was articulated and validated. And it was the first time Helen realised there were different forms of knowledge and ways of knowing – which could all be valued in nursing practice. In Table 3.1 we've drawn out how Carper's four types of knowing and forms of knowledge could be used in intensive care nursing.

Carper argues that all four ways of knowing are equal. However as McKenna (1997) points out, there are times or settings where a hierarchy of knowledge or knowing is more apparent; where empirics is more highly valued than aesthetic or ethical knowing. At those times, it's a struggle to successfully argue that ethical or personal knowing is of as much value as empirics. We've tried to capture that struggle in the example of the critically ill patient in the data extract about intensive care above in Box 3.1.

As new tutors in a school of nursing in the 1990s, Helen and her colleagues were introduced to Schön's (1987) writings on the *swampy* lowlands of practice and the *hard, high ground* of academia or research. This helped them in their teaching to balance empirical nursing (evidence-based nursing) and other ways of

Table 3.1 Carper's ways of knowing, forms of knowledge and nursing critically ill patients

Way of knowing	Knowledge	Nursing action
Empirical knowing – the science of nursing	Biomedical knowledge Pathophysiology Anatomy Fluid/electrolyte balance Blood gases	Clinical observations for homeostasis Fluid balance Nutrition
Aesthetics – art of nursing	Artistry of care giving Performance of care giving Human engagement – presence, intimacy, humanising touch Expert practice Decision-making Leadership	Emotional care Physical care of the body Patients and relatives experiencing care Looking cared for Being cared for
Ethical knowing – the moral side of nursing	Human rights Information giving for consent/autonomy Cost/benefit analysis	Team discussions of treatment plans Decisions about when to continue/discontinue treatment Decisions about nursing care
Personal knowing – known through reflexivity either by self or in teams	Emotional effects of nursing critically ill patients/family Emotional labour in nursing Knowing the other Personalisation of care Clinical supervision	Relationships with patients and family Relationships in teams Valuing of care delivery

knowing which students described in their clinical stories during teaching and personal tutorials. Schön's swampy lowlands allowed them to validate students' clinical stories and make sense of the messiness of their learning. Using Schön's approach meant they didn't disregard their personal, emotional, aesthetic and ethical learning journeys.

Lawler's thesis on nursing the body (1991) uncovered and validated the messiness of nursing knowledge and practice which is what students were describing when they came into college. And it helped Helen and her colleagues challenge the hierarchy of nursing knowledge which privileged academic knowledge over knowledge of practice, in this case the body. Of course nurse teachers need to be quite clear that some nursing activities, such as dressing wounds, require theoretical knowledge. Other nursing activities are not underpinned by evidence and rely instead on other forms or traditions of knowledge or ways of knowing. These could be empathic knowing, aesthetic knowing or knowledge about how to reflect and learn. As Allmark (1995) suggests, the type of knowledge associated with nursing practice should not be taught through theory, nor is it well represented in theoretical terms.

The knowledge of the practitioner is not solely theory but includes theorising to produce knowledge and knowing.

Another typology of knowledge Helen was introduced to at this time (the 1980s–1990s) was know-how (knowing how to do something – skills) and know-that knowledge (the theory of action – why you do something) (Manley, 1997; Miller, 1989; Rhyl, 1963) (see Table 3.2). As a new and inexperienced nurse teacher this typology was incredibly helpful as it made sense of her struggle in teaching know-that knowledge to students who seemed to find learning know-how easier. They seemed to find know-how knowledge more relevant to their clinical experiences. Perhaps Helen's teaching methods weren't appropriate to allow them to process know-that knowledge? Helen found students' preference for know-how knowledge unchanged as a researcher when observing student learning in the early 2000s (see Chapter 4): know-how and performance were important for students and many times they gave convincing displays of know-how learning in front of their mentors rather than know-that learning. It wasn't until much later when conducting an action research project using reflective practice in supervision groups that Helen began to understand how recognising a hierarchy of knowledge between know-how and know-that to explore tacit knowing could be liberating for midwives in changing their practice (Allan et al., 2015c). However, despite this reflection, Helen continues to find that know-how knowledge doesn't underpin nursing theory in the same way as know-that knowledge doesn't always underpin practice. So much knowledge and knowing in nursing is developed from unintegrated learning: it's split if you like. This is possibly because historically, know-that knowledge has been valued more highly than know-how in nursing theory; in fact the theories which have emerged over the latter half of the 20th century served to devalue practice knowledge to the nursing theorist's personal advantage. Here we're thinking of American nursing theorists who have built up followers through basing entire curricula on their theory and educating students through this theory (McKenna, 1997). Murphy and Smith (2013) are quite right – this ideological stance by adherents to specific theories hasn't benefited nursing.

Table 3.2 Know-how and know-that knowledge

Know-how knowledge	Know-that knowledge
Often unarticulated conceptualisations communicated by word of mouth or role-modelling	Articulated conceptualisations communicated as theories, e.g. Watson, Henderson, Leininger; evidence-based practice, i.e. pressure area scores, MEWS scoring
Based on personal experiences	Based on invented or discovered reality
For the purpose of:	For the purpose of:
Delivering care	Describing,
Making sense of challenges in care	Explaining,
Team work	Predicting, or
	Prescribing care

We've adapted McKenna (1997) to add that the purpose of know-how knowledge may also be to:

- make sense of challenges in care
- build cohesive work teams
- support newly qualified nurses and other learners into teams and routines.

As with all typologies, this typology (know-that, know-how) is a falsification of reality. In practice most nurses use both forms of knowledge, as we shall illustrate through the data we've analysed using Evans et al.'s theory of recontextualisation. McKenna (1997) argues that knowledge development may come from personal experience (phenomenology) and reflection on know-that knowledge which leads to local refinement of know-how knowledge. As McKenna (1997: 38) goes on to say, 'practitioners could bridge the theory–practice gap by being encouraged and supported to apply research and theory to their practice. In this way, know-how knowledge would be the conduit for putting knowledge into practice.' Thinking about knowledge within nursing in the work of writers like Manley (1997), Manley et al. (2009), McCormack et al., 2008; McCormack & McCance, 2010, Reed (2006a, 2006b) and Rolfe (2006a) has built a body of work which has provided the theoretical basis for practice theory as well as provided evidence of nursing developing practice theory. Our work complements this body of work by providing a way to understand and conceptualise how nurses rework knowledge or theorise in practice through the work of Karen Evans and colleagues, who are contemporary educational researchers and theorists. We agree with McKenna that nurses are active learners and can theorise in practice, using know-how knowledge in practice to construct new knowledge which informs know-that knowledge or theorising in practice. We don't think this happens as a result of applying research though. Our aim in this book is to show that nurses are far more active and creative in their utilisation of research and knowledge than just application of knowledge even where this is an active thinking application. Building on McKenna's ideas about practice theory then, we use Evans et al.'s (2009) theory of recontextualisation to illustrate how nurses actively rework knowledge rather than apply it. We argue that students and professionals *put knowledge to work*.

Putting knowledge to work – the theory of knowledge recontextualisation

Evans et al.'s (2009) theoretical approach to 'putting knowledge to work', developed further in Evans and Guile (2012) and elaborated for post-qualification learning in Evans (2015), reframes knowledge transfer by arguing that knowledge in practice-based disciplines is not merely transferred from theory to practice but recontextualised in different practice settings. Students and newly qualified practitioners learn actively to change and use knowledge rather than passively take knowledge from one area to another.

Explaining recontextualisation

Understanding the flows of knowledge in programmes involving substantial elements of work exposure, such as in nursing and midwifery, goes beyond typologising forms and features of knowledge. Evans et al. (2009) argue that the knowledge logics that underpin programme flows, and how knowledge is changed as it is 'put to work' across contexts of learning and practice in universities, colleges and workplaces, need to be understood to produce reworked knowledge that will be useful for practice. All knowledge has a context in which it was originally generated. Contexts are often thought of as settings or places, but contexts in our use extend to the 'schools of thought', the traditions and norms of practice, the life experiences in which knowledge of different kinds is generated. For knowledge generated and practised in one context to be put to work in new and different contexts, it has to be recontextualised in various ways that simultaneously engage with and change those practices, traditions and experiences.

Evans et al. (2009) have argued that recontextualisation is multi-faceted pedagogic practice, based on the idea that concepts and practice change as we use them in different settings. The original research has drawn on developments of Bernstein's idea that concepts change as they move from their disciplinary origins and become a part of a curriculum (Barnett, 2006; Bernstein, 2000) and on van Oers' (1998) observation that concepts are integral to practice and change as practice evolves over time and varies from one sector or workplace to another. These notions have been substantially expanded to embrace the ways in which learners themselves change as they recontextualise concepts and practices.

Four kinds or sets of practices of recontextualisation are significant:

1. Content recontextualisation – how knowledge is selected and connected in the programme design environment, for purposes of teaching and learning.
2. Pedagogic recontextualisation – how knowledge is reworked in the teaching and facilitating environment.
3. Workplace recontextualisation – how the interplay/interfusion of different forms of knowledge generates new knowledge in the workplace environment.
4. Learner recontextualisation – what learners make of these processes, over time and at different stages of their professional lives.

Putting knowledge to work in the programme design environment: content recontextualisation (CR)

The theory–practice relationships depend in part upon the ways in which knowledge has been 'codified' in accordance with the rules and procedures of specific, sometimes competing, disciplines and schools of thought that inform the field of practice. When curricula are created, this occurs through content recontextualisation (CR) – when knowledge moves from its original context of production (for example in the academic research community or an industry research and development programme) into the formal learning programme offered by a learning provider. This is a process whereby codified knowledge is selected, simplified, recast and made more teachable and learnable for the intended participants, as part of the programme design. This is not necessarily an entirely peaceful process as different interest groups hold allegiances to (a) different forms of knowing, (b) different disciplinary knowledge (physiology, sociology, psychology), (c) forms of knowledge (know-how, know-that) and even levels of theory (see Chapter 9).

In professional and vocational education, this content recontextualisation process entails the selection and organisation of disciplinary and codified occupational sector knowledge to meet the presumed demands of professional and vocational practice. Different knowledge logics complicate this process, as logical structures that move towards higher levels of abstraction and theoretical understanding interact with knowledge logics that rely on a series of practical, operational connections. Disciplinary knowledge logics rely more on forms of codification that provide principles for selection and recombination. Procedural and work process knowledge are less formally codified but may be understood as knowledge generated and developed in and through action in the complex dynamics of practice. Codification generally does not address relations between these two types of knowledge, which are partly distinct but also interacting and interdependent (drawing on Alderson, 2020). So practitioners involved with curriculum design must develop and agree criteria and practices to determine how content based on different forms of knowledge should be selected and combined to achieve programme goals. This content recontextualisation (CR) entails the first set of knowledge recontextualisation practices.

Putting knowledge to work in the teaching and facilitating environment: pedagogic recontextualisation (PR)

Once different knowledge logics have been connected in a curriculum, the focus changes to pedagogic recontextualisation (PR), the design and organisation of the teaching and learning dimensions of programmes. PR takes place as different forms of knowledge are organised, structured and sequenced into learning activities, options, modules, for the purposes of effective learning and teaching. Pedagogic recontextualisation practices involve teachers, tutors and trainers in making decisions about how much time and emphasis they want to devote to activities developing and connecting different forms of knowledge, striking a balance between time and freedom to engage with these forms of knowledge in their own terms while progressively focusing attention on knowledge use in specific areas of practice. These decisions are never technical matters; they are often contested. They are inevitably influenced by teachers', tutors' and trainers' tacit assumptions about what constitutes good learning experiences and worthwhile learning outcomes (Evans and Guile, 2012). They may also be circumscribed by the specifications set by professional or examination bodies and time available for exploration of topics according to tutors' pedagogic preferences is often a limiting factor and possibly a source of frustration. Academic nurses and practice-based nurses often disagree about the extent to which students need to engage with nursing theory. Reconciling conflicting views entails pedagogical recontextualisation practices, in which the challenge is to ensure that concepts and general principles are well understood and elaborated as work-based learning provides a series of suitably challenging 'test-benches' for the use of knowledge in action.

Putting knowledge to work in the workplace environment: workplace recontextualisation (WR)

Workplace environments fundamentally affect how knowledge is put to work, and they vary considerably in the nature, extent and quality of learning experience that they afford. Workplace recontextualisations take place through the workplace practices and activities that support knowledge development, and through the mentorship, coaching and other arrangements that enable new entrants to engage with and learn through workplace environments. These practices and supports are fundamental to undertaking standard workplace activities effectively and to developing the confidence and capability to work with others to meet and change those activities where the situation demands it. They allow learners to experience how individuals and teams progressively recontextualise concepts as they experience demanding practical situations and confront unexpected problems. This is a form of learning that is often triggered by the activity and the context. Knowledge recontextualisation takes place when:

- A student or newly qualified practitioner recognises a new situation as requiring a response and uses knowledge – theoretical, procedural and tacit – in acts of interpretation in an attempt to bring the activity and its setting under conscious control (van Oers, 1998).
- The interpretation involves the enactment of a well-known activity in a new setting: an adaptive form of recontextualisation takes place as existing knowledge is used to reproduce a response in a parallel situation.

And where:

- The interpretation leads the learner to change the activity or its context in an attempt to make a response, a productive form of recontextualisation takes place, as new knowledge is produced (Allan et al., 2018).

Knowledge recontextualisations are fundamental to learners and new entrants beginning to enact existing workplace activities, or working with experienced others to modify or change them in the face of unexpected occurrences or the need to find new solutions. These workplace recontextualisations are facilitated when workplaces create stretching but supportive environments for working and when learners expect, and are expected, to take responsibility for observing, enquiring and acting on what they learn. Learners, through a series of such knowledge recontextualisations, come to self-embody knowledge cognitively and practically. This is the start of a long-term process of personal and professional development that is difficult to detect, elusive of measurement and often appreciated only in retrospect.

What the learner/employee makes of it: learner recontextualisation (LR)

What learners make of these recontextualisation processes varies according to their personal characteristics and the scope for action that they have, individually and collectively, in any particular environment. Together with their prior learning and tacit knowledge, opportunities and affordances for learning may be unequally distributed (see Evans et al., 2004, 2006). Learner recontextualisation takes place through the strategies learners themselves use to bring together and put to work different forms of knowledge they have gained through the programme, through working with learning partners in college and workplaces and by observing, enquiring, and working with more experienced people in the workplace.

Learner recontextualisation is critical to the development of a professional identity. The theory–practice relationship is reflected in the interplay of professional and academic identities, and in the longer-term development of the new entrant as a knowledgeable practitioner (Evans, 2015). Thinking and feeling one's way into a professional identity is facilitated by such practices as engaging in 'learning conversations', articulating developing understandings and sharing perceptions of practice with others, being stretched through opportunities to work at the next level. Most importantly, the development of the learner as a knowledgeable practitioner continues beyond qualification: through mentorship, coaching and peer learning, and by reflecting, continuously and critically, on new ideas and experiences accessed through work and through wider professional and personal networks that extend beyond the immediate work environment.

Connecting the four expressions of recontextualisation.

Each of the four expressions of recontextualisation sheds light on some element of the challenges of connecting theory with practice and relating subject-based and work-based knowledge in the processes of professional learning and practice development. When connected, they offer a framework that can be used to analyse existing programmes, interrogate research and design new approaches (see Figure 3.1).

The framework in Figure 3.1 summarises and provides a simplified representation of the ways in which recontextualisation processes can combine in learning programmes. Knowledge from disciplinary sources is combined with occupational sector knowledge and codified practice-based knowledge, recontextualised through CR into the content of the curriculum or learning programme. Teachers and facilitators of learning develop teaching, learning and assessment strategies that recontextualise the content into activities to generate worthwhile learning processes and outcomes (PR), connecting directly and reflexively with work-based practice and the affordances of specific work environments through WR. Learners draw on their prior disciplinary knowledge and on their prior and current work experiences in the ways in which they engage with the teaching, learning and assessment strategies and eventually their new work roles (LR). These processes are facilitated when learners

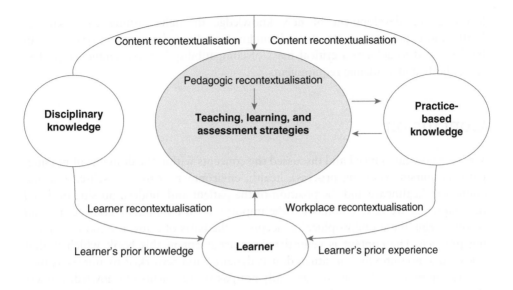

Figure 3.1   Putting knowledge to work framework

develop meta-cognitive strategies; and when learning partners work together to help the learners, whether students or newly qualified practitioners, to see connections and make sense of the whole process.

This theoretical framework has strong implications for professional practice. It means that the longstanding language of 'transfer' hinders rather than facilitates the search for solutions to the 'theory–practice' gap. Using the concept of recontextualisation explains the ways in which all forms of knowledge are tied to context (settings where things are done); and

- identifies what actions assist people to move knowledge from context to context
- identifies how knowledge changes as it is used differently in different social practices (ways of doing things) and contexts
- identifies how new knowledge changes people, social practices and contexts
- identifies who and what supports the recontextualisation process.

Putting knowledge to work to meet educational, sectoral, organisational and learner needs depends on greater use of recontextualisation practices across all teaching, learning and workplace environments as a way of maximising the integration of subject-based and work-based knowledge and developing strong foundations for knowledgeable practice. For example, the original research (Evans et al., 2009) has shown how the construction of multi-faceted, multi-level partnerships between colleges, organisations and workplace sites can embed knowledge flows in and across programme design, teaching and learning and the facilitation of learning in workplace practices. Recontextualisation can be assisted by the 'gradual release' of knowledge and responsibility to learners over time and in contexts of increasing unpredictability of tasks. Using 'Industry Educators' as knowledge brokers can support the effective use of workplace and professional resources for teaching and learning, and development of new knowledge through learning conversations. Furthermore, programme structures including coordinated assessment practices can be developed to achieve a critical mass of compatibility between employer, professional body and academic requirements.

Conclusion

We have now introduced and discussed the concepts within the domains of nursing: patients, nursing (nursing process), health, environment, care and self-care in the context of healthcare and the position of the patient and modern nursing outlined in Chapter 2. We have emphasised the importance of continually considering and reconsidering these philosophical concepts as the basis of critical thinking in nursing practice. The context is central to our argument in this book which is that knowledge is contextual or situated; it is dynamic and reworked by nurses as they theorise in practice. Nurses are generally not passive recipients of knowledge unless they are prevented from thinking or their conditions of work make thinking too difficult. As our argument in this book is based on the premise that nurses actively use knowledge in practice (situated knowledge) with knowledge learnt elsewhere (both academic and other practical knowledge), the context in which nurses think or theorise must be acknowledged. Our intention is to rework recontextualisation in nursing practice to understand how nurses theorise in practice.

Putting knowledge to work to meet educational, organisational and learner needs depends on greater use of recontextualisation practices across all teaching, learning and workplace environments as a way of maximising the integration of subject-based and work-based knowledge and developing strong foundations for knowledgeable practice. Original research by Evans et al. (2009) has shown how the construction of multi-faceted, multi-level partnerships between colleges, organisations and workplace sites can embed knowledge flows in and across programme design, teaching and learning and the facilitation of learning in workplace practices. Recontextualisation can be assisted by the 'gradual release' of knowledge and responsibility to learners over time and in contexts of increasing unpredictability of tasks. Using nursing mentors (industry educators in Evans et al.'s original description) as knowledge brokers can support the effective use of workplace and professional resources for teaching and learning, and development of new knowledge through learning conversations. Furthermore, programme structures including coordinated assessment practices can be developed to achieve a critical mass of compatibility between employer, professional body and academic requirements.

McKenna (1997), Avis and Freshwater (2006), Reed (2006a, 2006b) and Rolfe (2006a) all suggested an alternative approach to thinking about theory. We have briefly introduced such a theory here. Rather than presenting ways of bridging the gap, a new way of thinking is proposed to enable students to integrate their learning in what is currently a disintegrated learning context. This builds on writing on practice-driven theory and different forms of knowledge in nursing. The focus here is on *knowledge and theorising* rather than theory.

We shall return to theory and the theory–practice relationship in Chapter 8 after the following 'data' chapters, where we illustrate our argument that nurses *theorise in practice* by drawing on findings from studies of learning in the workplace where nurses and student nurses have reworked knowledge in practice.

It seems to us that nursing has for too long attempted to bridge the theory–practice gap through the wrong conceptual framework. The passive transfer of undigested knowledge only means that knowledge which is said to be useful and applicable in practice, in reality cannot be used in practice unchanged or unprocessed. This can be dispiriting as this undigested, unprocessed knowledge appears to be superfluous to practice and only useful for passing examinations. No wonder students become disillusioned or cynical and then reject theory and in the process, assert that they have no use for theory.

In the following chapters, where we draw on research data to illustrate how nurses theorise in practice, we shall focus on workplace and learner recontextualisation as this is where students and nurses put knowledge to work. The studies we've used to do this have focused on clinical learning with students and newly qualified nurses, clinical practice with fertility nurses in advanced clinical roles and management with senior commissioning nurses.

4

The studies

Chapter objectives

This chapter presents the studies on which we shall draw in the following chapters to show how nurses theorise in practice. They include:

- *The Leadership for Learning study*, which investigated how mentors and ward managers (nurse leaders) influence the ways in which student nurses learn in practice in the NHS post-2000 (Allan et al., 2007, 2011; O'Driscoll et al., 2010; Smith et al., 2010).
- *The Delegate study*, which studied newly qualified nurses' learning as they transition to managing patients in acute ward areas and (importantly) managing support workers (Allan et al., 2015a, 2016a, 2018; Johnson et al., 2015; Magnusson et al., 2017).
- *The PEGI study*, which investigated the professional experience of changing governance and incentive arrangements for the management of patients with long-term and complex conditions in health and social care (Allan et al., 2014; Ross et al., 2009). This study focused on interdisciplinary roles in mental health teams in the management of patients with long-term mental health conditions in the community.
- *The developing fertility nursing roles study*, which explored how fertility nurses in fertility clinics practice at an extended level in specialist roles when taking on medical tasks to care holistically for infertile couples (Allan and Barber, 2004, 2005).
- *The role of commissioning nurses or GBNs (governing body nurses) study*, which considered emerging new roles of senior executive nurses in clinical commissioning groups where direct nursing care is not the basis of the role (Allan et al., 2016b; 2016c, 2017; O'Driscoll et al., 2018b).

Introduction

We now introduce the studies we will use to illustrate our argument that nurses (and one or two other health professionals), no matter at what point in their career and across clinical settings, theorise in practice.

Leadership for learning 2008–2010

This study investigated how changes in nursing leadership roles have influenced the ways in which student nurses learn in clinical placements in the NHS. A summary of the Leadership for Learning study report is available at: www.surrey.ac.uk/sites/default/files/2018-04/4.USE-Survey-Final-report.doc. We focused on new leadership roles and their influence on student nurse learning, given the change in the ward sister's role during the 1990s and the introduction of mentors as the primary contact for students in clinical placements (DH, 1999). At the same time as these workforce changes were being introduced, major changes in nursing education occurred as a result of the introduction of new curricula in professional preparation programmes for nursing and the move of nurse education into higher education (see Chapter 2 for further details). Following these fundamental changes to nursing leadership roles and nurse education, a change in the public perceptions of nurses also crept into the public discourse with accusations that the move of student nurses into universities had rendered them 'too posh to wash'. There was media reporting of a general lowering of standards, including poor hygiene and outbreaks of serious infection, and the move of students to universities was blamed for this disastrous falling of standards (Scott, 2004). Concern was also voiced about students not learning in practice and a supposed overemphasis on academic learning despite a curriculum model which allocated equally shared responsibility for learning across college and practice settings.

Given these changes to ward management, nursing leadership and nurse education, the purpose of our study was to investigate the relationship between nursing leadership roles and student nurse learning in clinical practice – in other words, who is responsible for the leadership of student nurse learning in clinical practice?

Stage 1 included a literature review and stakeholder interviews with 10 leaders in nurse education. In stage 2, using an ethnographic case study research approach and three data collection methods (an online survey, clinical fieldwork and documentary analysis of written curricula) we collected data in four case study sites across England (see Table 4.1).

Our main findings showed that changes to ward management and nursing leadership roles in clinical areas and the move of nurse education to universities had profound effects for the leadership of learning in clinical placements for both student nurses and the staff who teach, mentor and work with them both in practice and in the higher education setting. Clinical learning was seen to be the remit of ward managers and although they were supported by practice educators, staff nurses, clinical nurse specialists, lead nurses or modern matrons, they maintained overall

Table 4.1 Summary table of staff observed and/or interviewed in informal, formal individual or formal focus groups across four fieldwork sites

	Site A	Site B	Site C	Site D	Total participants
Student nurses	4 2nd years (observation, informal interviews)	8 Individual 3 Focus group	7 3rd years (observation, informal interviews)	2 1st year student nurses (observation, informal interviews)	21
Lead nurses/ modern matrons	4 Focus group	1 Individual 3 Joint interview	3 Focus group	3 Focus group	60
Mentors	3 Focus group			3 Individual	21
Link lecturers	2 Joint interview		2 Individual	4 Individual	10
Ward manager	6 Focus group			1 Individual	37
Practice development nurses (PDNs)	6 Focus group		5 Focus group		66
Placement coordinator	1 in same Focus group as PDNs				1
Deputy director nursing	1 Individual	1 Individual			2
Senior Trust nurse practice education			1 Individual		1
Senior Trust nurse leadership			1 Individual		1
Practice educators		2 Joint interview 3 Focus group			22

responsibility for ensuring that the learning environment, including mentor training and support, was provided at ward level. However, due to an increased workload, including trust-wide responsibilities, their presence and attention had been taken away from the ward and students in many ways. Clinical learning appeared to be secondary to the drive for achieving clinical throughput and targets; this was typified by an obvious return to task allocation. The nursing process which was the predominant form of care delivery during the 1970s and 1980s, had now largely been abandoned due to the pressure to achieve targets. Task allocation in its new form of meeting discharge and bed targets and delivering trained nursing tasks (e.g. giving drugs) appeared to have been reintroduced and we observed a return to 'team' or 'sides' nursing (by which the work was divided into two separate 'sides' of the ward to which the nurses were then separately allocated) and a move away from patient allocation. This meant that students learnt on-the-job in much the same way as apprentices did for decades. Students felt that the learning they 'did' in college had little relevance to and was not valued by ward staff, whose main goals were clinical throughput or bed management and observing quality standards.

The delegate study 2011–2014

The Delegate study investigated how newly qualified nurses (NQNs) learned to delegate to healthcare assistants (HCAs) and the report is available at: www.surrey.ac.uk/sites/default/files/2019-11/AaRK-summary-report-2014.pdf.

Nursing is a profession for which demand is predicted to increase due to an ageing population and more people suffering from long-term, manageable conditions (NMC, 2018a). Caring for patients with long-term conditions has become as important to the health service as delivering new technological advances (House of Commons, 2017–2019; RCN, 2018a). The UK Government has made it clear that nurses will increasingly take up leadership positions in order to meet these challenges in future healthcare. Along with any projected future nursing roles, the current nursing roles have been subject to immense change over the last 30–40 years, as described in Chapter 2.

To meet competing demands on their time, registered nurses are increasingly delegating tasks to untrained healthcare staff due to rising healthcare costs, the need to maximise resources, skills-mixes, and the general expansion of health workers' roles. Delegation is the transfer of responsibility for the performance of an activity from one individual to another while retaining accountability for the outcome (Barrow and Sharma, 2019; Gravlin and Bittner, 2010). The term is closely related to other concepts, such as responsibility, accountability and authority (RCN, 2017; Weydt, 2010).

Delegation is seen as 'one of the most complex nursing skills … requir[ing] sophisticated clinical judgement and final accountability for patient care' (Weydt, 2010: 10). Delegation, patient safety and quality of care are unequivocally linked and poor delegation can provide fertile ground for errors (Eveleigh, 2018). Although delegation was not highlighted in the Mid Staffordshire Report (Francis, 2013), delegation is linked inextricably to clinical and nursing leadership, which was highlighted by the inquiry as flawed.

Delegation can be particularly challenging for NQNs but is under-addressed in pre- and post-qualifying nurse education (Hasson et al., 2013; Whitehead et al., 2013). This can lead to performance problems associated with time management (Eveleigh, 2018), inadequate workload distribution and insufficient supervision of delegated tasks, with associated implications for clinical productivity, patient safety (Neumann, 2010) and the patient experience (Cipriano, 2010).

The primary research aim in the Delegate study was to understand how NQNs use the knowledge learnt in university to allow them to organise, delegate and supervise care on the wards when working with and supervising healthcare assistants. This was a two-phase study which included a pilot to test a 'delegation tool' in phase 2 with NQNs on preceptor training programmes in three NHS hospitals.

Phase 1

This was a study across three sites. Data were collected using observations and interviews with nurses (HCAs and ward managers working at three hospitals). See Table 4.2, for full details of data collection from the three hospital sites, and Table 4.3, for profiles of each hospital site.

Table 4.2 Summary of data collected (November 2011 to May 2012)

Data collection method	Site A	Site B	Site C	Total
Observation of nurses	17 nurses 34 obs.	6 nurses 12 obs.	10 nurses 20 obs.	33 nurses 66 obs. (around 230 hours)
Nurse interviews	16	4	8	28
HCA interviews	6	2	2	10
Ward manager / Matron interviews	5	3	4	12
TOTAL (Interviews and observations)	61	21	34	116

From this first phase, we identified that NQNs need support during the transition from student to fully operational qualified nurse in the following areas: developing confidence; understanding role boundaries; accessing knowledge; developing communication skills; setting care priorities; achieving successful care outcomes.

Our research highlighted the significance of the changing roles and worlds of nursing for recontextualising knowledge as NQNs developed the critical skills of prioritisation, delegation and supervision of care within teams. The nursing curriculum in the three sites involved in the study appeared to prepare nurses only partially for the many demands of supervision, delegation and accountability in the modern staff nurse role. There was a need for increased focus on learning and support in this important area to assist NQNs to recontextualise their prior learning about a range of skills related to delegation such as communication, time planning, prioritisation among others.

Table 4.3 Overview of the three hospital sites which participated in the Aark study

	Site A	Site B	Site C
Ward specialties where participants worked	Emergency Admissions Unit (EAU)	Medical	Surgical
	Elderly	HDU	Respiratory
	Medicine	Surgical	Medicine
	Trauma	General	Gastro-intestinal
	High Dependency Unit (HDU)		General
	Surgical		
	General		
Approximate number of beds	700	700	450
Preceptorship programme	Yes	Yes	Yes

We argued that NQNs recontextualise theoretical knowledge in the workplace to emerge as competent and safe nurses but that they struggled to recontextualise knowledge and learning about delegation. How NQNs delegate to HCAs, and how they learn to supervise HCAs in carrying out those delegated tasks tend to be fairly ad hoc and contingent upon ward cultures and staff teams. This suggests the need for more structured educational/training support in development of the necessary skills. This may be in academic, practice or preceptorship contexts and might also involve simulated scenarios. In fact, simulation may help them to recontextualise or put knowledge to work in this key area of NQN practice.

This period of recontextualisation as an NQN is made even more difficult because it occurs in a liminal or transient and emotionally fraught space. There are support functions within the NHS to both recognise and support this liminal journey, most notably preceptorship courses but also informally in support shown by clinical colleagues towards the NQNs. Both sources of formal and informal support are highly variable across wards and hospitals.

Our final report detailed a framework to understand how NQNs transition through a liminal period of learning which involves three interrelated areas of development:

1. Organisational learning contexts: the context within which NQNs develop, recontextualise and use their knowledge.
2. Delegation in context: how the NQNs supervise and delegate care to HCAs and how the role boundaries are negotiated between NQNs and HCAs.
3. Learning processes: NQN knowledge development 'in action' and factors that support/hinder learning.

Phase 2

Drawing on the findings from phase 1, a preceptorship tool for organising, delegating and supervising care was developed to facilitate newly qualified nurses to focus on delegation. The tool was designed to be in addition to other learning, teaching and assessing approaches used within local preceptorship programmes for NQNs. The tool (Allan et al., 2018) comprised six areas for reflexive and supportive conversations relating to organising, delegating and supervising care of patients: Confidence, Role Boundaries, Knowledge, Communication, Care Priorities and Care Outcomes. Within each area were trigger questions to direct preceptor–preceptee conversations. The tool was produced in two formats (pocket-sized booklet and A4 sheet) so that the NQN can select the format best suited to that individual. An initial three-month pilot (October 2013 to January 2014) of the preceptorship tool was conducted with NQNs recruited from the three hospital sites. Each NQN was provided with an explanation of the tool and its purpose by one of the research team, and was given the tool in a choice of formats (A4 and booklet). It was envisaged that use of the tool would be supported within preceptorship meetings. The aim was that through use of this tool as part of reflective practice, the NQN would (a) find the tool useful in developing, organising, delegating and supervising knowledge and skills that are meaningful based upon their own experiences, and (b) recognise their own strengths and areas for further development. This would in turn expose the NQNs to opportunities to identify strategies for improved performance that would positively impact upon the quality of patient care provision.

After three months NQNs were individually interviewed, using semi-structured interviews, to explore their experiences of using the tool and individual NQNs' personal development in organising, delegating and supervising bedside care. Data were collected via telephone interview with 13 NQNs who had been given the pilot tool.

Among the 13 NQNs interviewed, some had used the tool and others had not. Non-use of the tool was often explained by systemic factors such as heavy workloads, insufficient time on the ward, and a perceived lack of a supportive infrastructure at ward and/or hospital level. A significant number of nurses described their non-use of the tool within the context of a preceptorship programme which they did not experience as meeting their needs. We concluded that those NQNs who were more orientated towards reflective practice, and who were in working environments which supported reflective practice, may have benefited from using the tool, particularly in the early months of transition from student to qualified nurse. Participants who had used the tool and found it helpful reflected that it had been of particular use during the early period of their transition from student to qualified nurse, especially in relation to delegation.

Different nurses had different attitudes to reflective practice and this also had an impact on their use of the tool. Several nurses were moving wards, planning to leave the trust and/or knew of friends who had given up nursing. Their observations offered insights into how inadequate preceptorship and support may contribute to the loss of NQNs either from specific wards/hospitals or from the nursing profession as a whole.

The professional experience of changing governance and incentive arrangements for the management of patients with long-term and complex conditions in health and social care – PEGI study 2006–2008

The PEGI study investigated how staff in the NHS were adapting to managing patients with long-term physical and mental health conditions in the community. In order to contain costs and manage increasing numbers of elderly patients living with chronic illness in the UK, there was a shift in the delivery of care from hospital to primary and community settings. To engage professionals and motivate them to change their practice in care of such patients, policies for social care and health professional curricula from 2007 onwards have emphasised that professionals should work together to promote choice, independence, and self-care closer to home (Glasby, 2006; Glasby et al., 2008; NHS, 2019). This situation is mirrored in other advanced health systems (Rudge, 2015) and continues to structure current UK health and social care policy (NHS, 2019). This shift in the management of patients with long-term conditions in the UK has been effected through the introduction of new governance and funding arrangements and, importantly, through changes to team structures and professional roles (Davies et al., 2005). Governance encompasses the tasks of management (decision-making and control of organisations) as well as the mechanisms for the relationship between organisations, and the social and political environment in which they operate (Glasby, 2006).

These policy changes meant that professionals with different educational and professional preparation had to learn to work together in new teams. Services can be commissioned as an integrated service with different providers (Cameron, 2011; Glasby, 2006; Glasby and Dickinson, 2008). However, working in integrated ways can be challenging for health and social care professionals (Baxter and Brumfitt, 2008; Cameron et al., 2014; Glasby, 2006; Hall, 2005). For partnership to work in the delivery of health and social services, West et al. (2004) assert that interprofessional team effectiveness must be predicated on factors such as organisational commitment, leadership, clarity over objectives, and coordination of the different and distinctive professional contributions (Cameron, 2011; Mackintosh, 1992; Poulton and West, 1999; West, 2004).

This was a three-centre study exploring the professional experience of changing governance and incentive arrangements for the management of patients with long-term and complex conditions in health and social care. Realistic evaluation was used to examine the interaction between varied mechanisms at play at an organisational level and to explore causal relationships between system change and key outcomes at a professional level. Pawson and Tilley (2004) argue that realistic evaluation is different from other evaluation methodologies as it seeks to understand how a programme works to effect change. This fitted with a desire to understand the human components of system change. The research team was interprofessional and led by an experienced health services researcher. Each site team consisted of a principal investigator and a co-researcher who collected and analysed data in each site.

The sites were local organisations for primary care, primary care trusts (PCTs); two cities (A and C) and one semi-urban location (B) were selected as representative of PCTs across the United Kingdom. In phase 1, service user reference groups (SURGs) were held in each site with 32 users with long-term physical conditions and non-psychotic mental illnesses to develop vignettes highlighting critical components of care from their perspective. These were used to inform the semi-structured interview schedules for managers (phase 1) and frontline staff (phase 2) (Ross et al., 2014).

In total, 32 managers and 56 health and social care staff were interviewed, working in newly formed teams delivering frontline care to people with complex physical or mental long-term illness. The teams included social service, district nursing and community mental health teams. Clinical staff working in these teams included community matrons, community nurses, occupational therapists, general practitioners, practice nurses, physiotherapists, community psychiatric nurses, social workers and specialist nurses. Interviews lasted between 30 and 70 minutes and recordings were transcribed verbatim and checked by the interviewer. The interviews elicited views on team performance, incentives, and the experience of managing care delivery in the new governance arrangements/partnerships and organisational change.

The findings of this large study are detailed in the final report which can be accessed here: www.researchgate.net/publication/228553551_The_Professional_Experience_of_Governance_and_Incentives_Meeting_the_Needs_of_Individuals_with_Complex_Conditions_in_Primary_Care_Conditions_in_Primary. The research identified a gap between the statements in policy which might be better viewed as aspirations, and the *on-the-ground* responses of professionals who are expected to enact policy changes and their motivations as they struggle to do this. A key locus of struggle is the formation of new multidisciplinary teams; it is this struggle to form new teams that was noted at the time and reported in a paper on emotional responses to policy change (Allan et al., 2014). In the following chapters in this book, we draw out the ways in which this struggle also illustrates how community nurses, both mental and physical health, recontextualise knowledge to use in different ways due to the new experiences of working in multidisciplinary teams. These professionals theorise in practice as a result of working with other professionals from different disciplines which forces them to identify what exactly their nursing role is and what nursing knowledge they draw on.

Developing fertility nursing roles 2003–2004

While fertility investigations and treatments are increasingly being undertaken by nurses in specialist practitioner roles (RCN, 2018b), the development of extended specialist nursing in fertility care has been contentious. More than other areas of medicine and nursing, fertility is a largely privatised field of healthcare. As a result, biomedical science and technological innovation have dominated this field of practice. Medical clinicians have been reluctant to 'allow' nurses to develop specialist roles in a rapidly changing and unevaluated field (Allan and Barber, 2004, 2005) and the nursing role, which is rather more holistic and thus difficult to describe, has not been easy to define (Allan, 2001; Allan and Mounce, 2015). Finally, private healthcare tends to be more conservative in respect of developing nursing practice and, as noted, a large amount of fertility care is delivered in the private sector in the UK and globally (Allan et al., 2009b).

In the private clinic we studied, nurses were responsible for managing infertile couples' investigations and treatment cycles with supervision from a medical consultant and an embryologist. They had a degree of autonomy to undertake what were previously seen to be medical tasks such as ovarian ultrasound scanning, egg collection, embryo transfer and sperm aspiration (Allan and Barber, 2005). Specialist practice encompasses the knowledge and skills of a defined field of practice whereas advanced practice focuses on a defined level of practice, rather than type or speciality of practice (RCN, 2018b). In addition, 'advanced practitioners are educated at master's level and are assessed as competent in practice using their expert knowledge and skills, have the freedom and authority to act, and make autonomous decisions in the assessment, diagnosis and treatment' (RCN, 2018b: 6). This was a study of one unit where nurses were undertaking these skills, which are not often practised even today.

We used an ethnographic case study approach in a purposefully selected fertility unit where nurses practised extended specialist nursing roles as a single case from the small number of fertility units where nurses practise such roles. We collected data using focused participant observation of nursing in the unit and semi-structured interviews with five nurses, one healthcare assistant, one doctor and three infertile couples.

The findings suggested that such roles positively affect nurse–patient relationships in fertility clinics by increasing the level of continuity experienced by both nurses and patients. However, nurses do not claim to be intimate or close to patients; rather they 'know a great deal about a small area of their lives'. From these data we argue that emotions in nurse–patient relationships in fertility units where nurses practise in extended specialist roles are managed through a form of knowing the patient, which creates a feeling of closeness but at the same time maintains a distance or safe 'bounded' relationship with which both nurses and patients are comfortable. We use these findings in the following chapters to show how nurses reframe the boundaries of ethical care in fertility nursing – that is, they theorise their nursing role to justify extended specialist practice to themselves, to other nurses and health professionals in the team. Drawing on previous work on chaperoning in women's health (Allan, 2005) and the devaluing of nursing in current marketised, globalised health systems (Allan et al., 2008), we argue that the role of ethical knowledge and ethical knowing is the basis of theory for practice for these fertility nurses.

Commissioning nurses programme of work 2014–2017

Globally, different health systems have made efforts to restructure to assure efficiency savings (Allan et al., 2016b). Restructuring has led to managerialist systems (Rudge, 2015) based on forms of new public management (Berg et al., 2008).

Clinical commissioning groups (CCGs) in NHS England are examples of this trend (Allan et al., 2016b). CCGs commission 60% of health services in England and the clinical membership of these groups was initially limited to general practitioners (GPs). Following pressure from the RCN (2012b), each CCG was obliged to appoint a nurse to its governing body to *shape patient-centred service delivery*. It was asserted that governing body nurses (GBNs) would bring expertise from direct patient care delivery to population level commissioning. GBNs would apparently draw on enduring nursing values to enable them to act holistically with a concern for care, compassion, dignity and safety (RCN, 2012b). This view of nursing being grounded in compassion (among other values) was of course strengthened by public discourse in the wake of the Francis Report (2013).

The RCN's view was that nursing leadership was essential to advance the aims of the CCG. However, what was meant by nurse leadership in commissioning roles was unclear. What evidence was there that GBNs' practice was (as the RCN claims) based on compassion and holism? How did a direct patient focus transfer to a population focus? The NHS Commissioning Board (2012), briefing on the role of the nurse on the CCG governing body tried to clarify what is expected from GBNs by emphasising their expertise in direct patient care which is somehow translated to commissioning services at the population level. However, it says little about what informs or shapes this translation. The NHS Commissioning Board identify two types of nursing role: the registered independent nurse member of the CCG governing body and the executive nurse embedded on CCGs with responsibilities for CCG activities. This lack of clarity and the divergence of roles had been highlighted by early reports on CCG activity (Allan et al., 2016c; McCann et al., 2014; Trevithick, 2013).

In some ways, however, traditional forms of clinical authority may no longer be relevant. In work on professional knowledge and authority, Richardson (1999) argues that the growth and development of the medical profession has been dependent on individuals maintaining their clinical knowledge base and scope of practice. However, a new form of public management is increasingly apparent within public services. Here the increased use of contracted providers introduces competition and with it a greater emphasis upon performance, output and accountability (Larbi, 1999). Lawler (2005) asserts that in these new forms of public management, the term 'leadership' is virtually indistinguishable from 'management', and that generalised management and leadership knowledge are valued equally, if not more so, than traditional forms of clinical authority. This is because new public management emphasises the intensification of work, the measurement of performance in service delivery and cost efficiencies. It predominantly identifies with private sector managerial techniques and ideologies where focus is on performance management, increased surveillance of work, oversight and regulation through inspection and audit (Berg et al., 2008).

This new public management in commissioning prioritises rationality, the creation of autonomous agencies and the devolution of budgets (Berg et al., 2008), as well as an increased emphasis upon performance, output and accountability (Larbi, 1999). Newly emerging public management roles are not based on clinical knowledge and scope of practice, even when being carried out primarily by clinicians (Latimer, 2014). The type of leadership promoted by new public management prizes governance over clinically based authority (Richardson, 1999). Traditional nursing values of caring, perception and compassion may be difficult to assert in a commissioning context which is dominated by a belief that subjective experience and job-related knowledge are less important than skills in general management (O'Shea et al., 2013). Traditional forms of nursing authority are not dissimilar to medical clinical authority as the NHSCC and RCN argue, i.e. their authority is based on expertise in direct patient care delivery. However, nursing is a gendered profession and, consequently, has struggled to assert an objective evidence-based practice to its authority rather than authority being based on subjective caring actions or a virtue script (Bliss et al., 2017). It has struggled with being viewed as clinically authoritative in Richardson's sense.

The aim of the small programme of work was to contribute to the emerging knowledge base around GBNs' practice; three research projects explored how GBNs work within CCGs. In 2015, we conducted an integrative literature review (Allan et al., 2016b); and the same year (Allan et al., 2016c) we conducted a focus group pilot study to generate questions for a survey conducted in 2016 (O'Driscoll et al., 2018b) with GBNs and nurses working in clinical support units; and then in 2016, we conducted an observational case study using non-participant observation of CCG meetings, informal and formal interviews with CCG members at those meetings and with other CCG members (Allan et al., 2017).

We have argued from our three studies on GBNs that in the context of CCGs, a nursing professionalism based on clinical and gendered forms of authority becomes problematic. This is because such authority is contested by members of the CCG and external stakeholders irrespective of whether it is aligned with clinical knowledge and practice or with new forms of management. Both disregard the type of expertise that nurses in commissioning embody.

We conclude from all these studies that there is an emerging but highly individualised practice of nursing in commissioning on CCGs.

The findings from three studies into CCGs by Helen and colleagues contribute to a developing understanding of the history of nurses' involvement with strategic roles in governance (Davies, 2003) and leadership (Butterworth, 2014; Latimer, 2014) in health systems. In this book we draw on these findings to argue that nurses working in commissioning, who don't actually deliver care, are reframing how we conceptualise nursing and the role of nursing theory. We discuss the traditional framing of nursing theory which is grounded in nurses' philosophical beliefs around the person, the concept of health, the societal environment in which the person or patient lives and the definition of nursing as an act of caring. We suggest that irrespective of where nurses work and in what role, we can observe nurses theorising in practice. We present data to show how nurses in these new, non-contact roles are theorising their new nursing roles. This theorising has produced tension both for individuals and for how they are perceived by their practice colleagues (Smith and Allan, 2010). The new roles of commissioning nurse are yet another development of nursing roles where direct nursing care is not the basis of the role. We discuss how the changing nature of a nurse's area of practice, whether it is still face to face with a patient, reframes our fundamental philosophical beliefs about the nature of nursing and how nurses in such roles might theorise in practice.

Conclusion

While the studies drawn on in this book are varied, what they have in common is our concern with the question of how nurses at whatever stage of their career (including student nurses) make sense of nursing, the changes in the forms of care they deliver and the context in which they're expected to deliver these new forms of care. In these studies, irrespective of how experienced or inexperienced the nurses might be, these studies show how nurses make sense of evolving nursing roles and the rapidly changing contexts in which they work. Their deliberations and struggles as they negotiate these changes are not helped by a lazy and convenient discourse on the theory–practice split; it is more empowering (and resolves the theory–practice split) for their professionalism to understand their deliberations as theorising in practice.

In the following three chapters, we draw on these studies we've introduced to illustrate two recontextualisation practices: workplace and learner recontextualisation. Our argument is that these recontextualisation practices which nurses engage in illustrate theorising in practice.

5

Theorising in practice through workplace recontextualisation

Chapter objectives

- Discuss workplace recontextualisation (WR)
- Introduce *activity* and *context* act as triggers of learning for nurses as they practise
- Draw on data from studies 1 and 2 to show how these triggers prompt learning in the workplace. We refer to learning in the workplace rather than clinical placements which is more routinely used in nurse education literature.

Introduction

There is a long history in professional and occupational learning of considering workers as lifelong learners (Vähäsantanen et al., 2017), although this is not common in the nursing literature. It may seem odd to refer to learner recontextualisation when talking about qualified and experienced, even executive nurses, as we do in this book. We do so because nurses are lifelong learners who engage formally in continuous professional development and informally in adapting to changing workplace practices, or organisational restructuring. The data in this book illustrate their commitment to lifelong learning. After all, a feature of professionalism is the ability to adapt to change; developing identities as a professional is evidence of the individual's ability to be agentic, and we consider this further in Chapter 7 (Vähäsantanen et al., 2017). While they form their professional identities early on in their careers (Bentley et al., 2019) many will choose to move to clinical specialisms and roles and therefore develop a further identity embedded in the new area of clinical practice. For many nurses, this will be part of positive career development. Many will be forced to move specialisms due to workforce reorganisation and restructuring and may find adapting to change difficult. Hence, we recognise that registered nurses are adaptable, agentic, flexible professionals who have developed lifelong learning skills.

Workplace recontextualisation

As presented in Chapter 3, each of the four expressions of recontextualisation (workplace, learner, pedagogy and content) sheds light on the challenges of connecting theory with practice and relating subject-based and work-based knowledge in professional learning and practice development. Learners draw on their prior disciplinary knowledge and on their prior and current work experiences in the ways in which they engage with the teaching, learning and assessment strategies and eventually their new work roles (LR). They make connections work for themselves individually as individual learners and develop a sense of the whole work process along with agency and identity as a professional. Learner recontextualisation (Chapter 7) is facilitated when learners develop meta-cognitive strategies and when learning partners work together to help the learners to see connections and make sense of the whole process.

Workplace recontextualisation takes place through workplace practices and activities that support knowledge development, and through the mentorship, coaching and other arrangements that enable nurses who are in situations which require learning (so we might call them learners) to engage with and learn through workplace environments. WR is also about the quality of the workplace teams and the types of and quality of the relational learning and activity in teams shaped by the clinical context. These practices are fundamental to undertaking standard workplace activities effectively and to developing the confidence and capability to work with others to change those activities where the situation demands it. These practices are the way individuals and teams 'progressively recontextualise' concepts in activity. This form of learning is triggered by the activity and the context.

Workplace learning in nursing

Of course, workplace learning in clinical settings has always been hugely important in nursing internationally (Forber et al., 2015) and continues to be so despite arguments around:

- placement capacity in relevant settings (Smith et al., 2010)
- a lack of a proper evidence base for practice learning hours (Barker et al., 2016)

- the role of simulated learning, its effectiveness and whether simulated learning can substitute for learning with real patients (Ricketts et al., 2013)
- the relative merits of short or long clinical placements (Levett-Jones et al., 2009) including other configurations of placement allocation such as 'hub and spoke'
- the varying quality of clinical placements, which depends on patient throughput and the 'busyness' of clinical areas, the relationships between learners, mentors and teams and the learning opportunities of particular placements as well as the ability, interest, and time for teaching among qualified staff (Cooper et al., 2015; Rebeiro et al., 2015).

Research into workplace learning in nursing has been focused latterly on competences rather than learning; with how nurses perform skills rather than the knowledge on which these skills are based and how both knowledge and skills are integrated through supported learning. Understanding how students and registered nurses learn to theorise in practice is another way to unlock our understanding of the complexities inherent in workplace learning and move beyond narrow concerns (even obsessions) with competence-based learning; and importantly, as the data from studies 1–5 show, to understand how nurses continue to learn until late in their careers and develop lifelong learning skills. Such understanding is crucial as society expects nurses to develop increasingly sophisticated levels of practice as healthcare systems evolve while at the same time employers expect nurses to become increasingly responsible for their own continuing professional development and learning. Our approach to theorising in practice demonstrates the limitations of this focus on competences and skills.

Workplaces fundamentally affect how knowledge is put to work, and they vary in the nature and quality of learning experience that they afford (Guile and Evans, 2010). WR takes place through the workplace practices and activities that support knowledge development, and through the mentorship, coaching and other arrangements with which learners/employees can engage and learn through in workplace environments. These practices and activities are fundamental to learners as they learn to vary and modify existing workplace activities or to develop the confidence and capability to work with others to significantly change those activities. Any worker must 'progressively recontextualise' concepts in activity. For example, the concept of blood pressure measurement takes many different forms in workplaces hence pedagogic, content and workplace contextualisation requires a range of supports to allow students to understand and thus theorise blood pressure measurement when confronted with patients who do not present with textbook symptoms.

How does workplace recontextualisation take place in clinical nursing practice?

Knowledge recontextualisation takes place in the workplace setting when:

- a learner recognises a new situation as requiring a response and uses knowledge – theoretical, procedural and tacit – in acts of interpretation in an attempt to bring the activity and its setting under conscious control (van Oers, 1998);
- the interpretation involves the enactment of a well-known activity in a new setting, an adaptive form of recontextualisation, which takes place as existing knowledge is used to reproduce a response in a parallel situation.

And where

- the interpretation leads the learner to change the activity or its context in an attempt to make a response; a productive form of recontextualisation takes place, as new knowledge is produced (Allan et al., 2018).

In Table 5.1, we illustrate how a nurse might demonstrate these three sets of knowledge recontextualisation in the workplace.

Table 5.1   Knowledge recontextualisation in a workplace setting – the IVF clinic

A nurse recognises a new situation as requiring a response and uses knowledge – theoretical, procedural and tacit – in acts of interpretation in an attempt to bring the activity and its setting under conscious control.	An example might be a fertility nurse recognising that a non-donor IVF couple seem anxious after a consultation with their doctor in the IVF clinic and may need assessment. Tacit knowledge here might be the trigger (the couple's body language) and the nurse draws on theoretical knowledge (familiarity with an anxiety and depression scale perhaps) or procedural knowledge (referral to the clinic counsellor). The new situation is the anxiety the nurse notices in a *non-donor IVF couple* as opposed to a donor couple who are required to have counselling about their donor IVF. Non-donor couples don't automatically get referred to the clinic counsellor. Note the nurse may draw on a wide range of knowledge and theory to recontextualise knowledge to bring an activity and its setting under conscious control.
The interpretation involves the enactment of a well-known activity in a new setting. An adaptive form of recontextualisation takes place as existing knowledge is used to reproduce a response in a parallel situation.	Continuing this example, the nurse realises that while she hasn't met this situation before, this non-donor couple are as anxious about IVF as a donor couple who routinely have access to counselling. They should be referred to the clinic counsellor even though this isn't usual practice. This is the adaptation which is provoked by the interpretation of new knowledge above.
The interpretation leads the learner to change the activity or its context in an attempt to make a response. A productive form of recontextualisation takes place, as new knowledge is produced.	As a result of this observation and the referral to counselling for this infertile, non-donor couple, the nurse begins to informally assess all couples in her clinic for anxiety and potential requirement for referral to counselling. She brings this up at a clinic meeting and all couples (non-donor and donor) are asked to complete a self-assessment for anxiety and depression at their first appointment prior to IVF. This is the new knowledge which changes both the activity (the assessment of IVF couples' anxiety and depression) and the context (the team meeting and orientation to the need for a broader assessment of anxiety and depression in new couples).

In the workplace, knowledge is embedded in activities which are themselves performed as routines and protocols using different symbolic and meaningful artefacts. An example here might be the 'patient observations' which are taken routinely at certain times a day according to a protocol (the scoring system called the modified early warning score or MEWS) using necessary but at the same time, hugely symbolic artefacts like the sphygmomanometer or the stethoscope. The key challenges include (1) learning to participate in workplace activities and use artefacts, and (2) learning to use work problems as a further 'test-bench' for 'curriculum' knowledge. This is facilitated when:

- workplaces create stretching but supportive environments for working and learning
- learners take responsibility for 'observing, enquiring and acting'
- WR is shaped by mechanisms or factors which either enhance or mitigate against WR happening: time/predictability, gradual release and enacting new knowledge.

Factors enhancing or working against WR

Gradual release, time/predictability and enacting new knowledge are factors or mechanisms which work across WR to enhance or work against recontextualisation.

Gradual release

In pedagogic and content recontextualisation forms, i.e. before and alongside the student learning in workplace or clinical placement, mentors or lecturers (those who are responsible with the student for planning learning) can carefully:

- sequence modules to build and integrate knowledge
- support learners to move between different spaces of learning; from the university to the working or clinical placement environment and back again.

Likewise, mentors and senior colleagues in clinical practice can structure learning activities for students to facilitate coherent learning. The gradual release of responsibility from teacher to learner involves learners being given incremental opportunities across two axes: predictability and time.

Time and predictability

Examples of time and predictability might be when students:

- strengthen and develop knowledge through extended time and exposure with familiar equipment, such as the stethoscope or wound dressing equipment
- are allowed to make mistakes in a controlled environment, closely supervised such as in the clinical skills laboratories or simulation, and increasingly, as students become more confident in skills in clinical practice
- feel confident when they move from predictable to more unpredictable tasks.

Feedback during a period of learning under supervision with a mentor or supervisor which is tailored to workplace and academic criteria further assists the learner in developing confidence to the point where the student is working under time and (un)predictability pressures of the workplace.

Enacting new knowledge

One of the biggest criticisms of the use of 'reflective' strategies in work-based learning programmes is that they are primarily designed to assist learners to gain accreditation or recognition for their existing knowledge, rather than to support them in generating and using new knowledge. The 'learning conversation' approach, which was an important feature of management development in the glass industry described by Evans and her team in the original work on *putting knowledge to work*, offers a way to escape this dilemma. Its key premise is that someone with extensive industry and facilitation expertise can design a conversational approach that not only recognises, but also expands, employee learners' knowledge and puts it to work. These conversations will assist the student/learner to put knowledge to work.

Learning conversations can be with formal mentors but also informally with key people occupying boundary roles for student learning such as (in nursing and midwifery) ward managers, senior colleagues, healthcare assistants, doctors, other healthcare professionals and fellow students or peer learners (as above in the example of the preceptor peer learning group). Activities for learning conversations might include:

- Shadowing
- Mating up
- Peer support
- Planning incremental responsibilities
- Debriefing that focuses on developing confidence in putting knowledge to work

Illustrations of workplace recontextualisation in clinical practice

We shall now use data from studies 1 and 2 to illustrate recontextualisation, starting with the following extract from study 2 which illustrates an *act of interpretation* leading to recontextualisation for a mentor who describes mentoring a student to do a medication round at lunchtime on her own but supervised by herself. She does this to allow the student to gain familiarity with the activity safely, i.e. with her remote supervision: in her words, to *build up confidence* in the activity (the medications, the computer) by bringing the activity under conscious control through doing something which is safe, i.e. lunchtime medications. But interestingly, she also describes through this act of interpretation, her own learning: bringing the activity of mentoring '*supervising a student undertake a medication round*' under conscious control '*allowing herself to tolerate the student do something she's assessed as safe*':

> Last year ... [a] student and she was absolutely brilliant and I let her do a lunchtime medication with my computer and I was feeding somebody and watching her doing it ... so in that way I trusted that student and she built up a confidence by, but you need to know if that student is confident and know what she's doing, I'll never ever let a student do morning medication without my supervision [working directly with student], absolutely not. Lunchtime medication yeah, it's more paracetamol and maybe some [thing] for the sickness if there is any but it's mainly the paracetamol so ...

Acts of interpretation can be activities which are facilitated in groups, as in another extract from study 2. In this NHS trust, newly qualified nurses (NQNs) participate in a peer learning group once a month. In the next extract, an NQN speaks about her learning in one of these groups. She talks about how she uses tacit knowledge *'having a little trick'* to utilise empirical knowledge *'when to give hypertensive drugs pre-operatively'*, which comes about by sharing learning with and learning from her peers:

> It was great being there with newly qualified nurses ... to go 'I just don't get it', 'which anti-hypertensive can you give before theatre', 'which ones [you] can't' and everyone else going 'ah, I've heard a little trick for that' or 'yeah, the way you want to think about that' ...

In the following example from study 2, an everyday act of interpretation is illustrated in the NQN's description of working in teams of NQNs and HCAs. The act of interpretation has led the NQN to learn that getting to know an HCA you work with and what she can and can't do will assist her in planning care as she learns to manage teams:

> So you try to know, try to know their limitation, what they can do and what they can't do.

While recontextualisation can seem like a fairly simple everyday action, i.e. getting to know staff you work with, it actually involves sophisticated human communication and judgements in acts of interpretation where the NQN or the mentor (above) brings what they know about the situation (the student, the medications, the potential for things to go wrong, the patients' condition, the plan for care, competencies of the staff she has working with her to deliver that care) into conscious thought through an assessment based on knowing what skills are needed for which task or activity and who can be expected and trusted to deliver those activities safely. In the following quote we can see how an NQN thinks or processes knowledge to arrive at this state of knowing, which she describes as *'[you] apply yourself well with doing what's important'*:

> And sometime I can be nervous but I try to learn... try to think of who I want to be like, like some mentor they are very calm, like very, you need calm to reassure the patients first because you cannot get nervous and you cannot panic on the actual thing so if you panic you stress out everyone and if you panic as well you don't know what's the next plan, you can't plan for the next, so we try to calm yourself, reassure the patient and apply yourself well with doing what's important, the next step is, so...

Acts of interpretation are smoothed by establishing a routine, as described by this NQN:

> I did struggle first, like maybe [a] month, two months nearly, until I got myself around routine and then, then it's gone better and better now, now it's, if we've got enough staff then if the staffing levels are good, then yeah you can get a job done, without too much stress and I can actually finish on time.

This NQN describes how seeing the *'nursing point of view'* through listening to patients helps her identify and assert her role as a nurse:

> Like multi-disciplinary team planning, so you can, you can raise your concern because you are the one with the patient most of the time so you know them better …
>
> **Yes.**
>
> Sometimes doctor[s] just see the medical point, they wouldn't see the nursing point of view so and some other issues the patient tell you quietly so.
>
> **Exactly, and I saw, I mean you seem to be very good at that.**
>
> We try to listen.
>
> **And I'm sure not all nurses are like that, you know with communicating those things.**
>
> I try to listen what they say and what their main concern is and their worries.
>
> **The patients.**
>
> The patients, their worries and so try to raise the concerns with the doctors, even though sometimes they, they just see only the medical point of view they wouldn't see other point of views, it's nice to go round with them and tell them your suggestion and they can decide how we can make a better plan for the patient.
>
> **And do you think generally they listen?**
>
> Yes, they do, yeah. I try to sometime you have to be assertive and advocate [for] the patient.

In the quote above, the NQN shows she's theorising in practice as she claims her unique nursing role through:

- listening to patients as they tell her privately what their worries are
- identifying these worries as different to medical concerns and as nursing concerns – as part of nursing and therefore her responsibility
- reframing patients' worries and communicating them to the doctors as a nursing point of view – again seeing this as part of nursing and her responsibility.

Her use of the phrases, *'medical point of view, nursing point of view'* is also interesting because it suggests that she is conscious of more than one viewpoint or worldview which are, until she reframes them in her role as patient advocate, in conflict and 'unseen' by the doctors: *'they wouldn't see the other point of views'*.

Sometimes acts of interpretation arose out of negative situations where learning hasn't been a positive experience. The student's act of interpretation in the following quote is to understand the reality of learning on a particular ward where she has felt excluded from learning:

> You know what am I doing here? I qualify in a month and not even drugs yet. I won't be able to do anything as a nurse. What have I done today? Caring not nursing; I know we have to do that, it's okay. Washes, beds, breakfasts, observations – but when they do drugs they should call me to look and learn. But they don't, so another shift wasted! (3rd year student, surgical ward)

Complexity of recontextualisation

As we've shown, recontextualisation is a complex learning activity partly because different stakeholders have different expectations and understandings of learning; it can be effected by the interplay between learner and mentor. Here the ward manager (WM) explicitly argues that knowing doesn't mean that all nurses (in this case NQNs) can nurse; in other words, that putting knowledge to work or recontextualisation is not always successful. She says this is down to the individual nurse's personality:

> ... you read sort of some of their work that they've done it always seem very and all very in depth and they know the knowledge, it's putting that knowledge into practice and it depends on the personality whether they're good at seeing what they're seeing and putting into practice what they're doing, everyone can talk a good speak about pressure area care but its whether they do it in practice.

The interviewer, Karen Evans, probes why these differences may occur in NQNs' performance. The WM replies that in her view, the difference in '*putting knowledge into practice*' is due to *personality* and *common sense*. However, looking carefully at what she says in this extract, she describes the NQN putting knowledge to work the next time the patient has a fall in the context of '*knowing who to escalate the incident to*'. This last statement suggests that the WM has recognised that by the second patient fall, the student has put her knowledge to work and is able to act appropriately:

> **KE:**   is it anything to do with the extent to which they go over what they've done and think about it and seek feedback and so on, is that an element of it at all do you think or not?

> No I don't think.

> **KE:**   it's just there or not.

> I keep coming back to sort of pressure care because they're, a lot of them are, it's obviously drummed into them about their sort of pressure area care and I just think you know, some of them do talk about it actually when you say 'well have you put them on a cushion?', well no they haven't done it, but if I asked the other girl she would have done

it because it's just common sense, but, I say where you've clearly said in your writing that you know, you would do it, so why didn't you do it, I don't understand that ... One of our girls – recently qualified, had a really nasty fall, a patient had a fall, cracked the back of his head, and I said to her 'you know what you have to do if there's a fall, who, who do you escalate it to, I know you've written about this because it was one of your concerns when you were training wasn't it?' 'yeah' she said, and I said 'and yet you never sort of escalate, you never sort of did the next step on from it, but you know what you have to do ... when I've talked to you now face to face you know exactly what to do but you didn't do it in practice and you know, and that sort of patient suffered sort of a head injury'. But now the next patient that had a fall, she did an absolute brilliant [escalation], so yeah, I don't know whether they think that you know, that people on that [academic] paper that they're writing about is a person today, you know [the] most frustrating thing about when you work with some students as they're qualifying and then you know what they're capable of but they don't seem to equate it to a real life patient.

She is probed on this by the second interviewer (CM) and this time suggests that it's not just (lack of) common sense that prevented the student from knowing how to escalate the fall/incident. She now says the student is not able to move beyond her academic knowledge to put that knowledge into practice when faced with a live patient:

CM: **and why, that's something in their training that?**

I don't know.

CM: **what is it?**

I suppose it's in their training, I don't know whether they don't get enough hands on, I don't, I have no idea, I don't really know why, why that is, because you, you know, you think back to your training, mine was very, very hands on training so it was completely different, we didn't have much of the sort of learning behind it and we wished we did so I don't know whether it is something about experience and just looking at patients I think, that's probably where you learn a lot from isnt it, I don't know, from their relatives and their patient themselves, I mean a lot of them can write very very, very good essays don't they and you just think 'oh come on' you need to think about it and put it to [work] as a patient.

She then goes on to suggest that the NQNs who are able to put knowledge into practice may have more experience with patients gained as HCAs, i.e. through having had more experience and developed confidence in workplace practices. In other words, by being exposed to practice experience and having had experience of putting knowledge to work.

Actually X was very good, she's got a good balance of what she writes and what she puts into practice, she, she's, you know, I think probably because she's been qualified a little bit longer when I got her so I think she had quite a bit of experience already under her belt, but she, because she's only been qualified I don't think all that long is it – less than a year ... She might have been March, yeah, anyway came with a little bit, maybe because she'd been a care assistant before as well so she just sort of seemed to sort of have a bit of both really.

As well as prior and continued exposure to clinical practice, putting knowledge to work may improve performance as continued experience of recontextualisation may assist in processing new knowledge in future instead of being *blinded* by new knowledge and situations. The ward manager in the following quote describes a scenario where having recognised this, the HCA might begin to use gradual release, and a learning conversation '*bring[s] them back to base*' to assist the learner to become more confident in future:

> ... so that they can direct them to some degree but in a nice kind of way, it's not telling them to do something but they will prompt them of what they need to do next to help them to manage the cares that are needed in that bay ... [NQNs] know that they have to some degree take the lead, shall we say because, although the student nurse will say 'I've done a lot of hands on care on the ward', when it comes to physically running a bay on their own, you do become very blinded very fogged shall we say because all you're thinking is 'I've got this to do, I've got that to do, I've got a million and one things to do' and 'actually my head's spinning already and I don't know where I'm going'. So sometimes the support workers will manage to bring them back to base and say 'right okay', say for example 'lady in bed one is self-caring, the lady in bed two we need to two of us to wash, the lady in bed three and four they will only need one for us to help them with personal cares, right okay, you do that one and I'll do that one and then we'll team up again afterwards'. We try to encourage that way of working.

Poor learning environments where recontextualisation struggles

The data from the five studies we draw on were collected between 2008/2009 and 2017 during a period of change and flux in the NHS (see Chapter 2). Common to all the studies are the references and descriptions of the busyness of the NHS; this is referred to by all interviewees and understood to shape learning in the NHS. Busyness was seen as detracting from learning across all studies but particularly in study 1 and recontextualisation did not figure strongly in participants' accounts in that study. Much of the learning seemed to the observer (Helen) to be about how to perform nursing rather than why a nurse was delivering care in a particular way. Helen observed that staff were orientated to allowing students to learn through doing but did not challenge them to expand their knowledge and skills or explore ideas cognitively. Indeed, much of study 1 data described when learning *didn't* take place. As this extract from Helen's field notes shows:

> Lots of learning what to do and how to be but not much why. It's as though embodied knowledge is hugely important – acquiring skills through doing – as one staff said today 'They'll have to be doing that soon'. (Field notes day surgery morning shift)

> Staff nurse and student doing drug round (2nd year student). Staff nurse letting student pour out tablets and give them to the patients; she didn't explain the drugs at all. She seemed to guide and facilitate the doing rather than understanding. At one point, she leant back, stretched her back and arms and looked for the world like she was bored. She didn't

teach or challenge ... at coffee, student said she felt 'taken care' of by her mentor who she always worked with. (Field notes day surgery morning shift)

While the student's feeling of *'being taken care of'* in her relationship during this drug round with her mentor was comforting for her, it appeared to Helen as if the mentor was role modelling how-to (procedural) and tacit knowledge at the expense of content or know-that knowledge which would be important on a drug round as patients need to receive the correct medications in the correct dose. This emphasis on procedural and tacit knowledge led to a few incidents where the researcher observed students caring for patients without knowing what their medical diagnosis was, as described in the following extracts from field notes:

The staff nurse allocated to work with the student that shift had not known what a [particular] scan was or how to explain a pulmonary embolus when asked by the student. So the staff nurse suggested we [Helen and student nurse] went up to see the scan. Helen then explained about the scan and what a pulmonary embolus was. (Field notes Accident and Emergency [A and E] late shift)

Student and I [Helen] were preparing a lady for operation; I asked student if she knew what the operation was; she didn't know and hadn't asked. Later mentor and student at the station looking at notes for the same patient going for parotidectomy that morning; mentor had arranged for student to prepare a patient and follow her through to theatres and watch the operation and care for her post-op. So again facilitative and meeting her identified learning needs. However she didn't check student knew what the operation was; so I asked the staff nurse in front of the student and she gave a brief explanation. (Field notes day surgery morning shift)

Helen's observations on the lack of know-that knowledge in the mentoring relationships that evolved as trained staff worked with students were validated in an informal interview with a ward manager, as recorded in this extract from field notes:

Sister told me that she thought students learnt how to do things but not why. 'We don't have the time. Don't know where they learn why'. (Field notes mixed surgical ward late shift)

In rather a negative way, these data show that the context in which learning takes place is hugely important and frequently, *it* was simply too busy to assist students to learn.

Factors which shape recontextualisation

It is known that certain factors can move recontextualisation from acts of interpretation to adaptive and then productive recontextualisation: time and predictability, gradual release and enacting new knowledge.

Time and predictability

Data showed how time and predictability were consciously and structurally planned to help the NQN learn. In the first quote, an HCA describes how systems like a structured handover are designed to help the NQN adapt and learn routine in order to enhance patient safety and effective team working:

> So that's like a structured one [handover], so it will prompt like the staff nurses to give a really good handover, a thorough handover, so most things should be handed over.

Other ways to facilitate time and predictability happened more informally through the performance of routine responsibilities as an NQN. Here an HCA in study 2 describes NQNs' learning triggered by an activity, i.e. being in charge for a group of patients and having to use the computer to keep accurate records. She describes NQNs gradually gained confidence through the performance of routine activities:

> They seem to be like, they're doing the same thing you know, took a long time on that, but I think it, I don't know, that's what I feel, that they just seem to be like lost on the computer sometimes and you know, it just takes them a while to do a certain thing but I suppose as they get more experienced they'll be a lot quicker at doing the care plans and stuff you know.

Time and predictability are therefore key to understanding how NQNs learn to recontextualise or put knowledge to work for themselves across different situations, as this ward manager explains:

> ... we always say it will take you all of that time for you to sort of get to where you think, you know – you won't think twice about picking up the keys or you know, taking the ward or whatever, so that's the nice thing about the preceptorship.

In another example, shown in Box 5.1, an HCA is frustrated that an NQN doesn't know how to take out a patient's drain on a surgical ward. She sees this as an example of how unprepared the NQNs are for practice. There's also some frustration that she's expected (because of her experience as an HCA) to show/ tell the NQN what to do. However here we can also see that intuitively the HCA knows that repeated exposure to the activity (removing a patient's surgical drain) is necessary to perform an activity in practice – in the HCA's words *'because I've observed ... I knew how to do it'*. She describes how repeated exposure has allowed her to feel confident enough to tell an NQN who has never done it before how to do the activity. Yet she denies the NQN the opportunity for the same learning process, *'she should know already'*. Sadly without repeated exposure, the activity will not become predictable and the NQN unable to move to unpredictable performance.

Box 5.1   Time and predictability

I was with another staff nurse who'd been here for a while as well and this newly qualified nurse was taking out a patient's drain and she wasn't sure how to do it, but I knew how to do it anyway because I've observed, I don't do that myself but we were telling her and I was telling her 'this is how you do it', I'm not even, I'm not even qualified to do that because I don't do that but when I'm telling her this is how you do it – I shouldn't be telling her like she should know already.

A little later in the interview she seems to acknowledge that the NQNs are learners although she'd rather they didn't rely on her as the more junior (and poorly paid) in the hierarchy:

Yeah, and there's always other people here that they can ask, but I just think that they need to know everything really about their patient and when they don't it's a bit [frustrating] cos they ask me … I don't know whether it's they're slightly embarrassed about asking what that kind of thing is, so they've come to me 'oh what is this', because they think I'm below them it doesn't matter if they ask me, rather than ask someone of their own level because they might feel a bit embarrassed I don't know.

Even seemingly well-known tasks and activities require time to produce adaptive and hopefully (finally) productive recontextualisation:

… they spend a lot of time on medication which I know I'm not qualified, but I've been here for three years and I know it don't take like 45 minutes to draw one [injection] fluid up, which some of our new ones are doing and it's not fair on us you know, we get, we get left with the confused, we get left with the risk of falls and trying to work all of that out as well as your daily jobs it's really hard, it is really hard.

However time and *predictability* as factors in facilitating recontextualisation are not always possible given the unpredictable nature of learning in clinical practice, as the WM suggests in relation to cardiac arrest:

The other big is that a lot of student nurses have never been exposed to sometimes is cardiac arrest, so in that situation that the nurses struggle because it is a difficult situation and it's not one that you have a lot of the time however now on the preceptorship course here they have started doing the intermediate life support so we are preparing for them for that situation in the future as well.

But the same could follow for any number of complex nursing tasks because recontextualisation is *dependent* on the placements NQNs have been exposed to in their programme:

... placements they've had within their training and where their exposure has been and you can certainly tell the nurses that are being exposed to places like A and E, Medical Admissions Unit, Early Diagnosis Unit, you know, surgical wards, because they know a lot of the background information and they can think about is that, should that patient be nil by mouth, have we filled in the surgical pathway, so a lot depends on where they've been.

The need for time and predictability is captured in this ward manager's description of NQNs' learning as a *'big learning curve, a big, big, learning'* which they don't have because they have two weeks from qualifying to learn. This lack of time has consequences, as she describes, in their drop in confidence:

... it's a huge difference isn't it from when the day that they qualified they have two weeks sort of supernumerary and then they're on the wards in charge of wards, right from the very early on, a big learning curve for them, I think it probably takes them about a year to really get their confidence built up again ... and it's just a big big learning thing.

Gradual release

NQNs were well aware of how activities, if unsupported or introduced too quickly in an unplanned way, could feel unsafe and prevent learning. In other words, how gradual release could enhance their learning, as this quote shows:

Do you feel you've had that all the time you've been here or?

No [laughs], at the beginning I hardly had, I haven't had a really good set up at the beginning, truthfully. They were always short staffed and I was sort of a supernumerary first three days, then day four I was thrown in to the bay on my own and on day six I was co-ordinating a ward with agency staff. And because my background is from the private hospital, I've never worked for NHS so it was difficult at the beginning. I wrote a statement obviously because I was not happy with the shift and anything could happen. And they said 'why, why don't you ring site co-ordinator?' Well my question was 'who is site co-ordinator?' I didn't even know there was a person called site co-ordinator because nobody told me.

NQNs' need for gradual release was well recognised by ward managers, although they acknowledged it could be difficult to implement. It also required investment and planning by a wide, supportive, clinical team (see Box 5.2).

Box 5.2   Gradual Release: Challenges for ward managers in busy settings

[NQNs] struggle with a change, the big change that we all have to go through from being a student to being a newly qualified nurse. And what they find is as soon as they put the blues on [registered nurses' uniform]

(Continued)

> they're ... all of a sudden people want them and they can't say 'I don't know something' or they're expected to give doctors answers.
>
> Time management we do have a practice trainer that will come and work with them, they do attend an in-house preceptorship for six months where they will attend one day a month and then also there's myself and we also have a co-ordinator X which is normally is band six or an experienced band five who are there to support them who are now supernumerary on this ward and that's something new that we've only implemented in the last month to be honest.

In many cases, gradual release is not always possible or planned for on a busy ward, as the NQN is at pains to describe in Box 5.3.

Box 5.3   Gradual Release: Challenges for NQNs in busy settings

And so, then when you started, could you tell me a little bit about those first months after you qualified.

For me, for me, my first month was really trying because I came onto this ward really, really busy ward, you've got to learn very fast, it runs at a very fast pace. And I felt like it was really [?? 08.19] for me and I felt like 'oh my God, is this what I was putting myself into' because, I mean the first, the first two weeks because you work with someone for the first two weeks.

Supernumerary.

Supernumerary, so that's fine, things going well, you don't know what you're, how it's going to be, when you're thrown out into it yourself and you've got to manage 13 patients, you've got to manage your own time and within those 7½ hours you are meant to attend to the patients, attend to the relatives, do your documentation, attend to the doctors as they need to know things about their patients, you know, [??] how it is, do your writing, do your medication, within those 7½ hours.

If this gradual release to exposure combined with support doesn't help the NQN perform to the level expected, then further support is introduced which places more burden on the clinical team. The skills NQNs struggle with most commonly cited by NQNs themselves, HCAs and ward managers are time management skills. The following WM describes the steps which are put in place for the NQN to acquire them: *working one-to-one, identifying gaps in skills and planning how to improve their performance.*

And when you say that 'in theory' and that some of them struggle with it, what do you do, how do you help them if they struggle with that?

The, we will work with them on a one to one basis and try to look where they are, not managing their time correctly and put action plans together.

And what would, what would be included in an action plan like that?

The action plan would look at the allocation of medications, how long it takes to do a medication round, how long it would take to do a ward round, what risk assessments they have to do that day, they would look, we would look at the overall care of a patient and whether there's some training needs more than anything because that [is] what it tends to be, training needs, to then free up some time for nurses to provide hands on one to one care with patients.

Despite the busyness and the challenges of transitioning from senior student to NQN, many ward managers recognise how important gradual release is to learning and successful transition. In the data extract in Box 5.4, a ward manager illustrates her awareness of the challenges NQNs face and how activities can be structured: *paced* to facilitate recontextualisation or learning to *forward think, forward plan*.

Box 5.4   Gradual release and successful transition

Ward manager speaking:

It's just physically learning the [computer] system and then the other thing is you know, a lot of training days are advertised on the hospital intranet. So it's learning how to and having the forward thinking, the forward planning to, to look on the learning development website as well to find those study days for themselves

Yes, it's a lot to begin with, that's why I think in the 3rd year student, they should be given some autonomy and their mentor should under observation let them manage to begin with one patient, then two patients ...

And would you expect that, them to be able to do that from day one or would it be?

No, no, no, no, I think it's unfair – no, not from the day one, even though they're 3rd year ... because it's a responsibility ... it has to be a really certain pace. You have to think constantly, have to think 'what's next, what's next'. So that's why I think they should be introduced you know, let them see how we work, and gradually preparing them for what's next and you say next week you could look after a patient, the following day two patients, and the following week perhaps, this is a middle of placement here I think, to get used to the environment and to sort of, we also have a lot of discharges, admission[s] and it's very fast and sometimes it could be a bit exhausting for us, never mind for a student who has a lot to take in to be honest.

Enacted new knowledge

A team approach to putting knowledge to work can be structured when the individual NQN works with a senior nurse who can probe and challenge the NQN:

> think that's another big learning thing for them really our walk round handovers with a good person that does it, a senior nurse that does it and just goes through it step by step and I think you know, and you question, why is their blood pressure like that, you know, and is there something that's happened, what are you thinking about their low blood pressure, are you going to sort of escalate that up and, I think that's another sort of learning thing really in the very early days really. (WM)

Here the NQN says she participates in enacted knowledge as she watches those nurses who are slightly her senior and listens to their tips on how to become more confident:

> **And how have you learnt to prioritise do you think?**
>
> Through practice, and practice, watching how other people do their thing and really through practice and asking and also watching how other people do it really. Because like for example I remember one of the girls telling me 'if you really want to manage for example in the morning when the doctors are doing their rounds, you could write what they, what they have decided about the patient then, because you're standing there with them, if you have the time scribble what they have written then if anything comes up like if there's any change you can add it to that'. So then you know you've done that otherwise if you leave it to the end then there's a possibility that you're going to forget what they have said.

The support for enacting new knowledge doesn't have to come from a senior nurse. The data show that HCAs are key members of an NQN's work team. HCAs described observing NQNs learning as they begin to make connections through workplace practices and activities:

> I mean sometimes you get, over the years you get into like a routine and you know what takes longer to do and I say you do get into a routine. But with newly qualified, it's like 'what shall I do first?' And it all depends on what patients you've got and what's happening you know. Well they do tend to get through it but a slower process you know, because they're not used to it. But they do fairly well and if they get stuck they do ask you know, others. (HCA)

However, NQNs don't always feel supported by their colleagues – as in this extract where the individual NQN was left on her own to establish a routine:

> I did struggle first, like maybe month, two months nearly, until I got myself around routine and then, then it's gone better and better now ... now it's, if we've got enough staff then if the staffing levels are good, then yeah you can get a job done, without too much stress and I can actually finish on time.

Adaptive recontextualisation

When the act of interpretation involves the enactment of a well-known activity in a new setting, an adaptive form of recontextualisation takes place as existing knowledge is used to reproduce a response in a parallel situation. While the following data from study 1 don't show the greatest supportive learning environment, they do show students are active learners who show adaptive recontextualisation. In at least two episodes of observation in study 1, it quickly became clear to Helen that the students she was working with were accustomed to sorting out their allocation of work including who they worked with. They enact well-known activity (allocating the work) in a new setting or parallel situation (each morning shift with new students).

> Morning shift had handover. The ward manager comes out of the office, then staff nurses, then two students trailing behind; allocation already done. Students look hesitant but then started breakfasts. I introduced myself and was told to go and find the students. Later that shift while having coffee with these students, the 3rd year student was angry about what had happened at the start of the shift 'you saw what happened? – we just sorted it out – the other student is pregnant so I took the heavy side. The staff nurses were already busy on the phone so we had to do the work, decide what to do. No-one supervises you.' (Field notes Gynae-oncology late shift)

> Very slow start to shift with mentor appearing slow to ask students what they needed to do or indeed identifying them as students who needed to work with mentors if present – my student said to me later 'I wait to see – is she going to sort me out? Obviously not! – Then I decide what I want to do and who to be with'. (Field notes A and E morning shift)

In the following extract from study 2, the NQN's active learning appears to be quite stressful for her. The adaptive learning is conveyed in her description of her existing knowledge '*First priority is to do my medicine round and then I take it from there really*', which she enacts in a new or parallel situation '*one particular day, we were so, so busy*'. There's a sense that she has an internal mantra to get her through stressful, new situations such as when it's busy '*the basics – medicines, observations*':

> First priority is to do my medicine round and then I take it from there really. There was one particular day, I mean we're so, so busy and I knew I wasn't going to get me jobs done. So I did my medicines, I did my obs[ervations] and then I got everybody washed and cleaned, and I couldn't get much more done than that, but I was happy with that because I'd felt that I'd done the basics, so it would be medicines first, erm, then, then obs[ervations], well then anything that needed doing in between, then obs[ervations]. And obviously, because on this particular day there wasn't anybody to do the washing, so I was going round, you know, doing them.

In Box 5.5, from study 1, a longer illustration of adaptive learning is given from Helen's field notes of a long piece of participant observation. The adaptation is shown in the student's reflection on a patient she has found emotionally challenging: in her saying '*We couldn't help. That's what I found difficult when I'm not in control. The other stuff is okay because we can do something.*' So the sacral sore, the repeated need to clean up the bed-bound patient were examples of where she'd learnt to recontextualise knowledge and become confident and adapt to new situations. Meeting the needs of a dying patient and doing an electrocardiogram (ECG) were aspects of the role she was continuing to struggle with.

Box 5.5   Adaptive recontextualisation – being able to reflect in practice

It was 07.45 on an early shift and a 1st year student was working with sister on a very busy ward. Helen offered to work with the student in one *'heavy'* bay.

... 2nd patient was confused, had kept the bay awake by shouting, smelt of faeces and needed a full bed bath. Student went to gather things we'd need and we started. The woman had a big sacral sore, necrotic and 'dirty' with faeces. The bed bath took about 45 minutes; it was hot, smelly, and difficult to move the woman and the student was unsure of herself. However the woman kept saying 'thank you' and looked better afterwards; she then went on to be incontinent of faeces 10 minutes afterwards. After two more bed baths and an assessment of a lady who'd 'gone off' (it turned out to be a trans ischaemic attack) and doing a set of observations and calling sister who did a superb mini teaching session, we staggered off to coffee. I remarked how tired I felt and joked I wasn't used to hard work. The student said she liked to be busy and hated being bored; gets bored with two–three hour lectures. Prefers mornings so she can be busy; she likes her mentor to show her once and then leave her to get on with things (as she doesn't like not doing). But if it's something like ECGs then she's scared of them and keeps asking to observe.

I then remarked I'd found the woman's sacral sore difficult to deal with – it was a long time since I'd seen one. 'Oh you just get on with it. I'd never seen anything like that before but I have now and it's fine. I just think if you can help someone, like we were, she kept saying we were, then that's okay. But before Christmas there was a man with legs that were very painful, they were falling apart and he was in pain. I couldn't do anything and I found that difficult. To see someone come in and then in a week, like that go downhill and die. We couldn't help. That's what I found difficult when I'm not in control. The other stuff is okay because we can do something.' (Field notes medical ward morning shift)

And finally, an NQN in study 2 reflects on learning in university and in placement and what facilitates learning in placement: firstly, she looks to the mentor for guidance but if the mentor isn't up-to-date, she actively ignores and recontextualises what she observes with what she's learnt in university in adaptive recontextualisation:

I try to learn the good skill that I want whoever like, in university they teach you, they guide, they teach you in the lot of very good lectures and they guide you – the books to read, those are very useful I think, those books are, and when they send me placement the mentors are, I try to learn from and [??], you try to learn the good things from mentor and like things you don't want to [??], you don't want to be like that, you don't learn.

Exactly.

So you don't, you try to learn from a book.

Almost like bad role models or ...

Yeah, so not that bad like a bit, not update practice, I want to take like [??].

And what can you try and describe what those good things are then that you try and pick up from the mentors?

Well some of them the mentor, I wouldn't say they are not up to date but like it depends.

Not up to date with what, knowledge?

Yes, like knowledge, the way we do things in the trust.

Productive recontextualisation

Where the interpretation leads the learner to change the activity or its context in an attempt to make a response, a productive form of recontextualisation takes place, as new knowledge is produced. In the following extract, in an informal exchange with a mentor in charge on a day shift who was working with a 2nd year student, Helen asks the mentor whether she liked mentoring:

I had dreadful mentors when I was a student and I swore I wouldn't be like that with anyone.

The mentor shows that she's changed the activity (mentoring) and its context (her relationship with the student, engagement and interaction with the student) as a response to her experience as a student. A productive form of recontextualisation has taken place, as new knowledge is produced to work differently as a mentor. The next quote shows another example of productive recontextualisation where an NQN recognises that the activity and setting of delegation have changed in her transition from student to NQN: 'delegating as a student and delegating as a staff nurse are two quite different things'.

And the management skills that you're developing, did you get some insights into that in the programme?

Yeah, we did but delegating as a student and delegating as a staff nurse are two quite different things.

Yeah, how would you say they're different?

They're different because it's, it's hard to delegate as a student, because erm, I did try it once and erm, they didn't, the support worker didn't like it very much. I did it in a nice way, and I think it's, not so much easier, but you feel like you, you've got more authority to delegate as a [NQN], not that I've, I've struggled delegating … delegating but you've got more authority as a staff nurse than you have being a student.

Even where the learning environment is poor, as in study 1, with fewer positive examples of workplace recontextualisation, productive recontextualisation was described as taking place. In the next extract (see Box 5.6), Helen has gone for a coffee break with one or two students who are interested in what exactly she's doing working with them. Helen's been working with them on the gynae-oncology ward, morning shift. The atmosphere has been quite sombre and Helen felt the students were perhaps being shielded from the distressful death of one of the patients. The students were distressed by the atmosphere on the ward. Productive recontextualisation is revealed in the 3rd year student's resistance to the possibly well-intentioned but clumsy teaching by a practice educator. *She reveals how she resents the learning activity of reflection and being asked to 'share' what a personal and painful experience has been. Her pain and anger are revealed in her descriptions 'until you explode' and 'I hate being asked "what have you learnt?"'* New knowledge is produced through her interpretation of her need to reflect alone or possibly in a small group unforced as occurred during our coffee break together.

Box 5.6   Productive recontextualisation in a poor learning environment

There were two young patients dying, one patient who'd had a total abdominal clearance and had come back to the ward in shock and was being resuscitated; the curtains were drawn around her and one of the Sisters kept going in and out. Neither of the students were looking after these patients.

At coffee with a 2nd year and a 3rd year student nurse, the 2nd year student asked me if I'd always enjoyed nursing?

I replied 'yes' but it had been difficult. How was she finding it?

'It's been difficult; shocking coming into nursing from school; the amount of work'.

The 3rd year then said that she found the 'stress and psychological [effect] builds up and feels heavy on your shoulders until you explode which is what I did the day before with the practice educator'.

A 2nd year asked me if other link lecturers (I had told her I taught as well as researched) worked with students. 'They're not here. Sometime in other areas they're useful; I had one in my first placement, a care home. Here the practice educator comes and.'

3rd year interrupts 'it wasn't reflection. It was should! Should! Should! Not helpful. He fires questions at me and I can't think. I hate being asked "what have you learnt?"'

2nd year 'I can't think quick enough and they continue to fire questions at me. We have reflection in college'.

3rd year 'Yes but there you don't want to share with 30 others. It's difficult, gynae-oncology and you can't share this (nodded towards the ward) with others. It's the emotions of caring for them, (nodded again) that gets on top of you'.

Conclusions

So do these data illustrating WR show that nurses theorise in practice? In our view, there's certainly evidence of thinking and reflection and as a result, adjustments to activities and practice in the acts of interpretation we've presented. The data show how nurses theorise about their professional:

- identity
- nursing roles and activities
- purpose, i.e. patient care and advocacy
- leadership built on teamwork, being calm and organised, establishing a routine, working with others.

The data also show their ability to manage ambiguity, complexity and conflict. The findings illustrate how these nurses, including ward managers, healthcare assistants, newly qualified nurses and students:

- thought about the reasons why they care in particular ways
- articulated to each other in handovers or in case conferences the rationale of what the nursing care is based on
- thought through ethical practice
- thought through their own learning preferences.

These data reveal how complex WR is and that, despite the busyness and almost constant state of change in the NHS, WR is a feature of work and learning. The NHS appears to sustain learning despite students feeling their learning needs are not always acknowledged and ward staff finding supervision of students challenging.

These data from study 1 show poor learning environments where evidence of knowing (know-how), tacit and procedural knowledge is present in clinical practice but know-that knowledge appears to be absent. However, even in these circumstances, students appear to learn and theorise through negative incidents as well as positive in response to challenging contexts of care. Whether these apparently ingrained habits of learning can be attributed to the ways in which the organisation explicitly fosters strong learning, foundations, dispositions and identities in early career nurses and the extent to which it is generated and sustained in the unique ecologies of learning and practice (Barnett and Jackson, 2020) of the NHS is a matter for later discussion (see Chapter 9).

We will now move to the data from studies 3–5 to illustrate other situations where more experienced nurses theorise in practice through WR.

6

Theorising in practice through workplace recontextualisation among experienced nurses

---

Chapter objective

- Using data from three studies, we illustrate how experienced nurses learn in the workplace at all stages of their careers

---

Introduction

In Chapter 5 we presented data on workplace recontextualisation from studies 1 and 2, which illustrated how student nurses and newly qualified nurses learn and theorise in practice. In this chapter, we present data from studies 3–5 on workplace recontextualisation to illustrate how experienced nurses also learn and theorise in practice and are lifelong learners.

The studies are:

- study 3 (interdisciplinary roles in mental health teams in the management of patients with long-term mental health conditions in the community)
- study 4 (fertility nurses' practice at an extended level in specialist roles in fertility clinics)

- study 5 (emerging new roles of senior executive nurses in clinical commissioning groups where direct nursing care is not the basis of the role).

Illustrations of workplace recontextualisation in clinical practice

In study 4, relationships with work colleagues inside the fertility clinic were particularly important for the fertility nurses in workplace recontextualisation as it was within the safety of the clinic with trusted colleagues that they felt able to develop their roles. In papers published from this study, we called these relationships as being facilitated or hindered by the *internal milieu* of the clinic and argued that it facilitated role change because nurses felt they were supported and that they had a real choice about undertaking new roles. The milieu could also be affected by the presence of doctors who were not sympathetic to extended specialist roles and at these moments, the *milieu* hindered nurses practising in these new roles. The support and training delivered in interdisciplinary training in the clinic as part of this *milieu* motivated nurses to accept new roles and increased responsibility for performing medical tasks such as egg pickup. Our field notes show that there were a range of ways in which nurses worked which demonstrated an integration of new technical skills with traditional caring skills – the recontextualisation of knowledge and the production of new knowledge or theorising in practice. As observers who were also nurses, this entirely nurse-led team seemed revolutionary. We argued that this way of working changed the dynamics in procedures because of nurses' knowledge of both positions: that of the doctor or nurse performing the task and that of the nurse assisting the doctor and caring for the patient. This is described in the following extract in Box 6.1 where the nurse describes working and knowing each other as nurses during procedures. It illustrates an act of interpretation by the nurse of putting knowledge to work in a new way which fosters new team dynamics.

Box 6.1   Fostering new team dynamics

The main carer is the person who's taken the patient through from the waiting room because she's spent longer with that patient. Her role is to observe, watch, hold hands whereas the person who's operati[ng] can't do that, you can't do everything, you have to have an awareness of what's happening but of everything, what's happening in the lab, what the assistant needs to do, what the other nurse is doing, what the husband's doing ... you have to have the whole picture. The nurse who's looking after the patient really has that as her main focus and while she concentrates on the task, her focus is the patient. We know how each other works and perhaps I can suggest something to the other nurse without them thinking 'I'm being told what to do', you know.

This act of interpretation is developed further in the interview as the nurse explains how awareness of both positions enables the nurse undertaking the medical procedure to perform the procedure differently from a traditional nursing or medical position, as the nurse suggests in the following quote:

Interviewer: Do you feel the environment between doctor–nurse or nurse–nurse scenarios is different?

There is a difference in that they do the same job, just as well as each other. The nurses tend to talk more during the procedure. Explain to patients what they're doing. If somebody's jumping with pain, they tend to stop, give more sedation and then start again. I've noticed [my colleague] does that now more often! (Laughs).

However, what became apparent was that nurses felt a need to justify why they had taken on these extended specialist roles. At the time of data collection, the research team was struck by how taking on new roles prompted the nurses to reflect on their identity as nurses and justify their new roles as nursing. In the first extract, the nurse is anxious to retain a nursing identity in the face of possible criticisms that their extended, specialist roles makes them into *mini doctors*:

There's no way we are mini doctors. These are areas we are specialised in and we have more knowledge in these areas than a lot of doctors have and will have unless they work in the field full time.

And for another nurse, any new procedure becomes an extension of her nursing role. Thus she is able to affirm her happiness in undertaking a new role. In so doing, she theorises in practice about nursing and what it means for her and her colleagues:

And it is somebody that they actually know ... it's an extended role but I'm quite happy giving that sort of care, perhaps a little bit more than treating it as a procedure to be done. It's a part of, it's one investigation of a number that I would be doing [for that patient].

How personal this theorising was for this nurse is shown in her explanation that such transitions while acceptable and even expected, should not be forced on all nurses:

I think it's important that people aren't forced into doing things that y'know.

Many of the nurses in studies 3 and 5 were taking on roles and activities which are not traditionally associated with nursing. However, as they undertook new roles, they appeared to want to justify them in relation to a perceived core nursing attribute (often caring). In so doing, we suggest they are theorising in practice.

In the following extract, the governing body nurse (GBN) Sheila draws on knowledge and experience about ward nursing to justify her GBN position as a full-time executive nurse working as an elected member on a CCG. She theorises about her role as a GBN nurse by citing what she sees as nursing actions and in doing so aligns her executive role on a CCG with a ward nurse's role. For Sheila, the aim of both roles are to help the doctor. She puts her knowledge of nursing to work to do this (jokingly initially), to show how the GBN role is an extension of the ward nurse role.

> Sheila describes her role as executive quite a few times during our time together. Then at one point early in the observation, Sheila pauses to answer the phone, telling me afterwards it was a doctor on the line. She tells me jokingly that 'the role of the nurse has always been to help the doctor'. I ask how she defines her role compared to the GPs on the CCG. She describes her role towards the doctors as offering 'guidance and support' and that it is 'no different to being a nurse on the ward'. (Field notes)

Sheila claims that in her GBN role, she '*is helping the doctor*' and it is '*no different to being a nurse on the ward*', even while her role is an *executive* one. She is putting knowledge to work and theorising about her work as a GBN and its core values and attributes; in doing so, she justifies her role to her audience and perhaps herself.

Sheila continued to describe her role as a GBN at a second meeting with Helen – it almost felt like persistence. She clearly didn't want to be perceived as corporate and (in her eyes) evasive; on the contrary, she wished to be patient focused and honest. This then can be seen as her definition of GBN nursing: a patient-focused, honest executive which for her seems more in line with the ward nurse described above perhaps:

> I reflect to Sheila that she seems to interact differently with [the] trust lead than other members of the CCG team. She explains that when the duty of candour was being discussed, she 'sparked up [because] how do you make a discussion of contracts about patients?' She says that many of the other members are endlessly corporate and impenetrable. [She feels that] when she asks them questions, their response is evasive. Whereas, the trust lead provides clarity and honesty. For example, if there are risks attached to a situation, she will acknowledge these ... Sheila explains that she receives leadership training from NHS England. Her mentor asks her what motivated her to work on a CCG. She explains she was inspired by her values about patient care. Her mentor urges [her] to be true to her values, which Sheila considers has sustained her personal integrity. (Field notes CCG study 1)

Sheila's views about the GBN role are shared by other GBNs we interviewed and illustrate a sense of isolation for other senior nursing directors and managers. The chief nurses Sheila talks about are chief nurses who work in (provider) NHS trusts (community and acute) leading the provision of care, for example a chief nurse of a local hospital or community mental health trust.

> Provider chief nurses don't always understand about commissioning or the intricacies of commissioning, therefore [they] think that it is a bit of a mystery ... but I think a lot of it is personal – now, at this point in time, it's about personal credibility.

And again in this quote where the GBN sees herself and a director of nursing drawing on each other to succeed as nursing leaders – in her view their roles could be mutually dependent for their respective success:

> Despite tricky conversations about quality, I'd be nervous if I didn't have those relationships because I get assurance about quality to enable me to speak in front of say, patient groups. And directors of nursing need me because otherwise they'll be talking to a contracts person.

What becomes apparent later in the field notes when Sheila is again observed by Helen is that she sees herself as an executive who is also a nurse; she is focused, good at chairing, but attentive to individual contributions from those at the meeting. So while her activities might be very different to a ward nurse, her style isn't – she's attentive and assertive much like a ward manager who is in charge of a ward round. This style of leadership seems very different to that perhaps jokingly described earlier in the first quote above as supporting the doctors:

> She opens the meeting by referring to the action points from the previous agenda. She swiftly directs the team through the action points, asking for definitive outcomes 'we will consider that point closed'. Although she is focussed, I notice that she uses positive affirmation, always thanking people for their effort after each point made ... The content and the mood is executive. She is attentive but assertive, asking that amendments to the minutes are made in time for the next meeting. None of the others object but acquiesce to her leadership. (Field notes)

A second GBN described acts of interpretation as she explained her role to Helen during an interview. Tessa had taken a different route into the role and had a different motivation. Tessa was a practice nurse who on completing her BSc Nurse Practitioner programme then realised she was interested in strategic health policy planning and the nurse's role in policy making. She describes her interest evolving from her immersion in work as a practice nurse while studying which led to a gradual awareness of how her knowledge from her BSc informed her practice and constructed new knowledge. The interviewer asks her where her interest in service redesign comes from and she gives a clear example of WR where the effects of the BSc Nurse Practitioner *opened her eyes* and interacted with her work as a nurse: '*when you work in practice, you see what works well*':

> **Were you always strategic, did you do anything else before then or what was it in the course that?**
>
> I think it was, I did a project about how you can redesign sexual health services for children, for young people, and I started thinking, actually you know what, I'd be quite good at doing that, and looking at. Because when you work in practice, you see what works well and what doesn't work so well and where potentially you can make changes, and make the patient journey a lot smoother or just nicer. So, I don't necessarily think that I was that strategic focused until really I did my degree, really opened my eyes to looking at things from a different level.

The claims that Sheila and Tessa make about the GBN role being a natural development for a nurse, being similar to the ward role, is shared by other GBNs we interviewed who, in describing a nursing voice which would hold the commissioners to account, were theorising about nursing and the value of nursing to commissioning:

> [Nurses] were on the board to hold the professional responsibility and to advise the governing boards and they had a very strong nursing voice.

> [We] bring a consciousness of patient need to every decision whilst at the same time having a strategic overview of the wider population we serve. The secondary benefit to the CCG is that of the 'nurturing qualities' of the nurse to a developing, new organisation.

Although some GBNs in the study felt that it wasn't a nursing voice as such but a voice which challenged medical power:

> In my case it does not make a specific nursing contribution – it does however provide a non-medical and an 'unconflicted' clinical voice. It provides challenge and scrutiny on clinical strategies and an overview of quality and safeguarding matters. Importantly, the role also contributes to multi-professional strategic planning.

In Box 6.2, there is an extract from study 3 where nurses were being integrated more closely into interdisciplinary community mental health teams, and the nurse recognises a new situation (a reassessment for a post-natal depression) for a particular patient in an act of interpretation.

Box 6.2　An act of interpretation in recontextualisation – personalising an intervention

Yeah, I mean I think, you know, the classic might be I feel maybe that it's time to start on medication, um, and they're still, you know, feel maybe they don't want that and I would always support someone as long as possible. I had a lady recently who had post-natal depression, but it was complicated by also some of her life experience. And we went for about a year without any medication and, you know, she was, she was getting a little bit better, but it would be up, down. And she began, I felt, you know, in my opinion I felt that, you know, she wasn't getting any kind of stability to really kind of feel that she was feeling better long enough to really reap the benefits. And so eventually, you know, I said I felt that maybe we should be thinking about [a] trial of that. It took a long time, but I think it, you know, it, she did in the end decide that that's not what she wanted to do but, as I say, it was a long journey, but obviously with somebody else, who are very, very unwell, you might be having those discussions earlier on. (Community mental health nurse)

The following extract describing extensive service redesign and change was commonly expressed by our participants in both studies 3 and 5 as they recognised new situations which required learning:

Well, my role now, it has changed very recently in August but I work solely in primary care now which means that I triage patients who are referred from the primary care setting and I then decide on their pathways of care ... I think until August we did, we did part primary care, part secondary care and now in this team we are unique because this is the only team. All the nurses only work in primary care. (Senior community mental health nurse, primary care)

The words 'we are unique because this is the only team' seem to be important here in describing her act of interpretation, recognition of a new situation at work, and later she went on to describe how unsettling change and thinking differently are:

I think it is difficult ... because it's a completely new concept, it's taking a while for us to grasp it, so I ... It is difficult for the users of our service to grasp it and it's a case of sort of working with them to help to understand that it is a good thing, because it clearly creates a lot of anxiety. (Senior community mental health nurse, primary care)

Again later in the interview, she describes how her thinking and *rethinking* of her new role was difficult and led to anxiety, perhaps because (as she emphasises) she'd been working in the same way for *many, many years*:

But I suppose the difficulty was, we had to deal with our own anxiety first before we could help them with theirs, because it's ... for all of us, and those of us who have been in mental health for many, many years will be used to working in a certain way. All of these new ways of working do initially generate quite a lot of anxiety ... It's about having to completely rethink how you are working ... But these new ways of working do take quite a lot of thinking about, they do take ... You have to think... you have to leave aside what you have been used to thinking about it and how you have been used to thinking, and you have to sort of side-step and think well, OK, if we have to do that, how can we do it, how do we do it? (Senior community mental health nurse, primary care)

Complexity of recontextualisation

Adapting to change and thus adaptive recontextualisation, or rethinking in the quote below, was described as occurring in teams by several participants in the PEGI study – study 3. This process of rethinking as nurses adapted to new situations had a knock-on effect on patients which added to the complexity of individual nurses' acts of interpretation. In other words, nurses' theorising had at its centre patient wellbeing (Box 6.3).

Box 6.3 Adaptive recontextualisation and patient wellbeing

In this team [we] have gone full-time into primary care, which means we had to hand over all our secondary care caseload to other members of the team or they had to be discharged or ... [our life] was difficult. That was difficult ... (Community mental health nurse)

You know, people [patients] you have been working with for many years, have got a very good rapport with and people that you can spot in an instant if there's some change in their mental health or whatever, and we had to let them all go. So it was a huge adjustment both for us, for the nurses, and for the patients we were working with. But what it also did was it put quite a burden on the rest of the team ... (Mental health social worker)

And, you know, there're a lot of working and supervision with that as to what patients needed ... what these patients had, where they needed to go and all this kind of thing, so there was a lot of work. (Community occupational therapist)

But again, it was about rethinking what we were doing and how ... do we need any added-on different thinking, you know? (Manager, team leader, community mental health)

So certainly over the last three years for the nurses primarily, but also for the rest of the team, there's been huge adjustments to make because of these initiatives. (Senior community mental health nurse, primary care)

Significantly, the healthcare professionals we interviewed in studies 3 and 5 were in the midst of adapting to new roles and new teams brought about by structural and policy change within the health service – specifically, around the changes to commissioning (study 5) and changes to the organisation of long-term physical and mental health conditions in the community (study 3). Although they didn't describe themselves as learners, indeed they were all experienced nurses, they were in new situations where they had to learn to adapt to new working conditions and structures and new teams. This had the advantage of making their learning and theorising in practice more obvious to them as they described their struggles to adapt to new expectations and ways of working. Another feature of the study 3 data is that the staff we interviewed were not only nurses: they included occupational therapists and social workers working in new interdisciplinary teams. We have included data extracts from some of these other healthcare professionals as their struggle with new ways of working, their learning and theorising mirrors the nurses' struggle and was synchronous with it too as we collected data. Additionally, this synchronous theorising about the nature of their work questioned the claim that each profession had a distinct body of knowledge, which we will come back to in Chapter 8.

Workplace recontextualisation in study 3 was strongly shaped by external factors in complex ways such as threats of redundancy, reorganisation, relocation and restructuring or redesigning services and teams. The nurses we interviewed had a sophisticated grasp of the social structures including policy which constrained their professional work (see Box 6.4).

Box 6.4 Workforce reorganisation and workplace recontextualisation

I worked for two and a half years in the PCT and I could just walk back in their office, I could close their door and walk to the person's desk and talk to them. Now I have got to ask two or three or four people to find out who it is, and when I find them, they won't know what I am talking about. (Social/home care services manager)

The XXX structure is a top-down structure; that means that [xx] as director, he is employed jointly by us [County Government] and the PCT, and below him, he has got joint health and social care service managers, and health and social care team managers; half of whom are employed by health and half by us. In other words, its 50 : 50 funded ... so the management is joint but the teams they manage are still functioning separately. (Social/home care services manager)

The main issue I do have at the moment is that we have a Director that doesn't listen ... he's employed jointly by health and social care, but he's doing what was traditionally two roles and the expectation of the county council is that he's an Area Director like all the others but in reality his job is so much more complex than the others, so he's got to flit between the two and he doesn't have the time really to spend in each area. (Social/ home care services team manager)

Redundancy due to reorganisation and restructuring was another external factor which shaped workplace recontextualisation:

A lot of people are in doubt about their jobs and my experience has been that there's probably more disruption for us. (Director community services and service manager social/home care, joint post between health and social/community care)

These system reorganisations also affected some nurses' sense of their place in the system and how their work linked to others' in the same organisation and thus how to understand and theorise their work in the context of others and the patients they cared for:

[It] was better in when worked in social services ... in health, I don't think we had time to look at policies in detail. We might be told 'there is a change to a process' because of

> a policy but we wouldn't link it ... we wouldn't really be made aware of the whole thing. (Specialist nurse)

Trying to make sense of policy was further complicated by the impact of organisational change on organisational structure, which was seen as poorly aligned in terms of providing coordinated care for patients:

> It's incredibly confusing, it's ... We struggle with it, there's not a single member here that doesn't struggle with how the services are set up and how to access them and how Joe Public manages sometimes, the vulnerable Joe Public. (Mental health community nurse)

There were many examples in the data of healthcare professionals feeling stressed due to reorganised or increasing workloads, feeling bombarded by initiatives, and being near to giving up, and thus of a lack of recontextualisation or theorising as events overwhelmed them:

> I don't know if it was the end of last year or the beginning of this year, where I felt if I heard one more new initiative, I thought I was just going to give up because I just couldn't cope with any more. (Mental health community nurse)

Another community nurse described feeling 'rushed':

> I'm always rushed and going onto the next job and may be patients actually ... notice ... you know, that little special 10/15 minutes that you would sit with them, sort out the problem. (Social care services team manager [nurse])

A mental health social worker described the changes as having made time for reflection disappear:

> Because you need time to think and reflect and make sure that everything is clearly explained. Which does take time and I think that's the problem, you don't have time anymore. (Community mental health social worker)

Nurses described confusion due to rapid changes, half-implemented changes, and new patient referral pathways:

> I find some of these care packages very fragmented. And it's, to maybe get a social care package it's very difficult for me to initiate that or instigate that. It has to go through a whole referral process which is laborious and tedious and repetitive, so that makes that very difficult. And also accessing even within our own trust the therapy services, to enable people to stay at home. I find the system very confusing and if I find the system confusing, I am sure most other people do as well because I have worked here for a long time. (Community nurse, physical illness)

While service reorganisation was a significant (negative) factor in shaping the interviewees' experience in study 3, at least one interviewee was aware of other structural effects on her learning and professional practice (see Box 6.5).

> ## Box 6.5   The ability to reflect on the wider picture for recontextualisation
>
> I know that in America they do a lot of intensive visiting with enhanced families and vulnerable families and there's a sort of general service for everybody else. We are leaning towards that, but we're just so stretched that we, that I feel often that I can't give enough time to my enhanced because I'm still having to do the mundane stuff.
>
> So what would you say were the major, and you'll ... the language because you will have heard it in your degree, but the major philosophical shift, if you like? I mean in the policy for you?
>
> Um, I don't know. I think maybe this trying to prevent rather than cure, trying to get in there first rather than trying to mop it up afterwards. I think that's probably the biggest shift. Um, but sadly, some of the things that have, we've had to let go of are those that give us the best tools to know what to do. For example, antenatal visits, we used to visit every new mum who was having a baby for the first time and make contact with them, meet them, get to know who they are so that when you go in post-natally you get a bit of a feel for how they're doing. And we just, well, in other parts [of the county] they haven't been doing them for ages and it's something we feel quite passionately about, but we just actually it's one of the things that's had to go. (Health visitor)

Structural changes then had effects on WR at the level of thinking and conceptualising need and therefore how nurses theorise patient need and their role:

> It's a bit like Social Services, their threshold has changed. I mean they brought in, um, there used to be either they were enhanced with us or they were on a child protection register, there's now a kind of bit in-between now when they're a child in need, so there's a plan for them, but they're not on the, um, they're not as part of the child protection plan, so there's kind of this extra category, but that impacts on our work because often we're the ones that are holding the ball for that. Yes, they're involved in it. So again, thresholds are moving all the time, people are getting more difficult to get into because everyone is thinking 'Well, we've only got this much service, so therefore we've got to make the criteria this.' And that's what has an impact on the clients I think. (Health visitor)

Factors shaping workplace recontextualisation

Factors which shape WR for student nurses, NQNs and the fertility nurses in study 4 in clinical placements (time and predictability, gradual release, enacted knowledge) were not observed in studies 3 and 5. Perhaps this is because (a) nurses do not habitually think of themselves as learners when they have career experience, and (b) they are not seen as learners when they are required to learn because of redundancy, reorganisation and restructuring. Therefore their transition to new situations and/or roles is not planned either by themselves, by their organisation or by their new colleagues. Rather, in studies 3 and 5, recontextualisation was shaped by external factors in complex ways such as threats of redundancy, reorganisation, relocation and restructuring or redesigning services and teams. In study 4, however, transition to new roles and the learning that ensued was carefully planned.

Time and predictability

In this extract from study 4, the lead fertility nurse describes how the unit has developed an interdisciplinary training protocol for ultra sound scanning among other procedures which all staff have to undertake. It involved repeating activities, having a mentor, being assessed and repeating a skill until the assessor is satisfied you are competent. This approach of repeat exposure over time and demonstration of predictable competence facilitates putting knowledge to work: as she says, '*They may have the academic knowledge but academic knowledge isn't necessarily related to dexterity.*' To develop dexterity, practice is required.

You also have a role teaching doctors in their new role in the unit?

Yes assessing their scanning ability. Basically, if they have a problem with me assessing them, they take it to [consultant] because I have a responsibility to my patients in my care and the unit and I won't allow anybody unsafe to operate without saying something to them. So they have to take it really I'm afraid! I wouldn't allow them [to] operate without being safe on myself, so why should I allow them to do it unsafely on a patient? I think doctors are trained differently, see one, do one, teach one and we have gone to great lengths to develop these protocols and say that you have to do this training and do a number of scans before you can do egg collections and to be supervised and why should it be any different for doctors. They may have the academic knowledge but academic knowledge isn't necessarily related to dexterity ...

She goes on to say that dexterity isn't enough for understanding at a deeper level: time, repeated immersion and being comfortable with unpredictability are essential to assessing which treatment or investigation is needed for which couple:

... anybody can be trained to do procedures, egg collections, and that's not the critical thing. The critical thing is understanding what you're doing. And that only comes with time by seeing different scenarios but you have to use your brain every day, you can't go onto autopilot, you have to think about what you're doing, that's what makes it enjoyable for me. Because no two individuals are the same, no two couples are the same. Okay, a lot of the treatments are standard but you have to assess whether that standard treatment's suitable for that particular couple in front of you. That's part of the enjoyment of the job.

Gradual release

In the following extract the fertility nurse (study 4) describes how she practised her skills gradually building up confidence:

> I think it took approximately, everything was little bits by bits, after I did so many of one thing then I could do it on my own if I felt comfortable, um there's still lots of areas where I don't feel comfortable such as scanning, but everyone's really good and they'll [skills] come.

Enacted knowledge

Many of the fertility nurses described learning conversations which were held in structured time with the lead nurse in the unit:

> **yeah, so you just call on people when you need extra support?**
>
> Yeah, and every once in a while I'll meet with Heather and go through with how I think I'm doing and what she's noticed, if I've improved or if I still need to work on certain areas, quite regularly.

Like some of the NQNs in study 2, Sheila recontextualised by thinking through her role and her growing confidence in what she was doing through an enacted conversation with herself and then me as the researcher. As she says below, CCGs are not valued by sectors of the NHS they work with and she obviously felt under pressure to justify her role; much like the NQNs as they learn to manage, to delegate and to organise work in bays. As the NQNs think that the focus of their work is perceived negatively by their colleagues, so too Sheila perceived her work as misunderstood by colleagues. The extract below shows how sensitive Sheila is to criticism (implied or perhaps explicit) of the GBN role and how she puts her knowledge of her role to work to enact knowledge, with the interview as a form of learning conversation (with herself as she'd obviously been thinking about this problem before I arrived to meet her) which facilitated recontextualisation:

> Met Sheila at 08.30 in town.
>
> She got me a coffee and I asked her how she was. She immediately said 'she was in a grump' and then said why: she'd been out for dinner the night before with a new director of nursing at a local acute trust who had 'no idea of primary care or health problems CCG was addressing' and yet was dismissive of CCGs. These acute trusts 'recruit to type' and probably are what they need. But thinking about effectiveness in health, she was probably more effective as she dealt with populations rather than a director of nursing who dealt with a tiny population in comparison. (Field notes)

Adaptive recontextualisation

Despite the complexity and burden of adapting to new processes, the nurses in study 3 clearly described adaptive recontextualisation:

> ... we would aim to be spending 45–60 minutes with patients on a visit, unless it's giving medicines or unless they are saying, 'I don't want you here for an hour, it's my evening, thanks very much.' I think patients get much more time with us than they would if they were on the ward for instance. (Community psychiatric nurse)

For one nurse manager, adaptive recontextualisation was described as she thought about how she was helping her staff to adapt to change:

> If you want people to work together, get them to talk to each other. It's probably saying really things will be better – putting names to faces and all of that kind of self-system stuff works very well. (Senior mental health nurse)

In a different approach, a manager of a team of professionals, working with people with physical conditions this time, described another form of adaptive recontextualisation where he focused with his staff more on performance or as he describes it, re-skimming:

> We're actually going down ... re-skimming these individuals and helping them to work through some of the ... through supervision, clinical supervision, peer supervision, really sort of sitting down and finding out what is it, what is the cause.

Fertility nurses also described adaptive recontextualisation (see Box 6.6). In this example, a fertility nurse in study 4 describes how each clinical encounter with a couple is not just a task, i.e. to give an injection (similar activity) as an extended specialist practitioner (new situation); it becomes an assessment of a couple's emotional state as well as their physical response to the treatment.

Box 6.6   Recontextualisation – responding to multiple triggers in the nurse–patient encounter

Say you're doing an injection, you're not just doing that, you're asking them how they are and you're getting a bit of two way conversation going that enables you to pick up on any other problems which are there. So it's not just an injection, they've come for information, to build up a relationship with you. Whereas I think doctors see that as a task. There's no point if you've got a couple who are very nervous, who are not feeling familiar with medical terminology, it's a waste of time giving every little bit of information. It's a waste of time. We need to get critical things across which are critical to their next stage of treatment. They don't need to know everything although there are some couples who do want to know everything. And we need to interpret very quickly really when we meet a couple, what information they need and why. And I might spend their first visit only talking a little bit about IVF, I know I've got to get that information across at a different time, but I think it's trying to assess the level of information they need at that time which is the deciding factor, what each couple needs. They don't want to be 'talked to' they want to be 'talked with' ... I think that's what['s] important.

Productive recontextualisation

Acts of interpretation allowed the nurses in study 4 to articulate the benefits of their new roles and develop a narrative of the role changes; we called this a moral narrative as the changes were often justified by the moral need to improve patient experience and comfort. They argued that their new roles had led to a more relaxed atmosphere during clinical procedures and consequently improved team dynamics, as described in this example of productive recontextualisation:

> The way we work now there's always a third person in the room. There's a big overlap of roles and sometimes the doctor or nurse will point out to the patient and the partner the screen. There's a lot of three way traffic going on between the operator who is talking to the patient and the nurse assisting and it's not separation of roles at all.

And here's another example of the production of new knowledge developed from previous learning and applied in a new situation (Box 6.7). The new situation is a different health system in a different country, yet the nurse is able to draw on previous knowledge – *reiki* relaxation *techniques, therapeutic communication* – to produce new knowledge as she practises in an extended nursing role as a fertility nurse assisting a couple during egg collection.

Box 6.7   Productive recontextualisation in new roles

… when I was doing my training we did quite a bit of psych, psychiatric nursing cos when you do your training in Canada you do all the areas you don't specialise … um, I did work on a psych ward for a while so, therapeutic communication you do go back to it … and use things like that. I hadn't done anything like hypnosis but we have done Reiki and healing touch in the school … so the same signal idea, just getting somebody to relax and get more comfortable during egg collection.

And do you think that knowing you helps that process cos that's an awful thing to have done to you isn't it, how d'you think they benefit from knowing you at that time?

Cos they've trusted you all along through their treatment and you've done all their scans and done all their appointments so there's already that trust there and they know that no matter what happens you're gonna be there and you're the one giving them the drugs and you're the one really that's gonna have the most of the control.

These interview data were not only examples of productive recontextualisation. These nurses were used to articulating narratives of their new roles, which was a way to communicate what they did to nurses and medical colleagues in other units; often in the face of resistance. The nurses we interviewed were aware that the unit they worked in was unusual; the nurses were among a handful of fertility nurses performing these procedures in the country. These extracts also show productive recontextualisation where production of new knowledge, *'we're all on an equal level'*, developed from previous learning about ways of working – *'It's not like our consultant is letting you do this and I'll do it whether I'm happy or not'* – and applied in a new situation *'empowering us to make our own decisions'*.

> There's an open culture. It's not like our consultant is letting you do this and I'll do it whether I'm happy or not. They accept that the days where we were told what to do and you do it even if you don't agree, they're gone.

> I think the dynamics within the team itself is important because we all get on very well together. We're very different but we seem to gel and there aren't any tensions between us. We've all been in theatres and the way surgeons behave ... we don't have that attitude and we're all on an equal level.

> The consultant [who supported the development of extended specialist nursing roles] was radical and didn't care what the establishment said. He was independent. He was very good at building people up, empowering them. He was very good, empowering us to make our own decisions but he was there if we needed him. He trusted us enough to get on with it.

This encouragement was based on trust within the clinic and it was observed that this trust was absent outside the clinic:

> There's a lack of trust that nurses experience from doctors because they don't think nurses have the academic background ... some doctors dismiss nurses as not understanding.

The nurses and the doctor interviewed were aware that, while they might view developing the nursing role as a natural extension of specialist practice, others outside in the fertility field did not. They perceived the external nursing and medical milieu as hostile to, and distrustful of, new nursing roles. The following extract is from the lead nurse in the unit, who had been the first nurse to undertake sperm aspiration in the UK:

> Whenever I do presentations on my role, you get either people saying 'ooh, that's really good but we're not allowed to do that' or they feel very threatened by it because they think people will expect them to do the same. Initially when our consultant asked me to do pickup, I said no because the climate [outside] wasn't right.

There were two aspects of these data which surprised us. The first was the extent to which the doctor also felt the need to *'keep quiet'* about these role changes and the multi-professional teaching programme she had begun to develop. The second was the fragility of the role change and how, in certain situations, for example working with locum doctors, nurses retreated from their new roles. The data suggest that professional communities can exert a pressure, perhaps unseen, around issues related to changing roles and consequently relationships between doctors and nurses. As the lead consultant says:

I think it's well known within the fertility nursing community. It's not well recognised within the medical community. I certainly don't hide the fact but I don't go out of my way to talk about it. I think probably because of an unconscious anxiety that many clinicians would be unhappy with what they would see as nurses doing essentially doctors' roles.

And another nurse reflects on their need for support in a possibly hostile professional field:

It was knowing someone else had done it first and had got approval within an NHS Trust. That gave us the confidence that we would be able to get through the loopholes to actually get on ...

This suggests that productive recontextualisation is dependent on a supportive and facilitative context for learning. In the case of the fertility nurses in study 4, their productive recontextualisation depended on the presence of a positive working environment which their medical colleagues controlled to some extent.

In Box 6.8 is an example of theorising in practice, productive recontextualisation, where an occupational therapist working closely in a team of nurses introduces a new activity (being authoritarian, taking patient to GP and then to hospital) in a new situation (self-harming which is threatening a patient's safety).

Box 6.8   Recontextualisation in occupational therapy

I had a client who, um, a very kind of long-term lady and actually I was her care coordinator for about ten years and she was somebody with a long history of very, very severe self-harm and she cut herself a lot. She also inserted lots and lots of wires into her arm that were really a time bomb in terms of the possibility of septicaemia. At the same time I knew that that was the only way that she coped and without that she might commit suicide or something more serious.

So there's a part of you that engages with accepting that she's doing that and she's deliberately infecting the wounds and, you know, she's expressed a belief that if she could just have her arm amputated everything would be alright.

Um, and it came to a point where, you know, and she would verbalise, she would say to me that, you know, she wouldn't want any treatment, she wouldn't take antibiotics if she had an infection then, you know, one day she came here ... I thought she might die, she was in so much pain, she had a huge abscess. You know, so you kind of, I just, you know, I said 'We've got to go.' You know, you become quite authoritarian. 'I'm taking you to a GP now.'

(Continued)

> We went to the GP and he said 'I can't deal with this, you'll have to go to the hospital now.' You know, and you find yourself kind of on the one hand for me I felt I was doing what was common sense and humanitarian, but at the same time, although she wasn't resisting, it was she'd expressed to me already a belief that she didn't think that's what should be happening.
>
> Um, and it's things like that that are on the edges of, you know, should we actually, if, because she said to me she wasn't going to accept treatment for it, do you then start to invoke the mental health act? But there's no provision in the mental health act actually to provide somebody, you can't provide physical treatment under the mental health act, so we had, you know, there was all sorts of debates and, and so that's where there's no, you know, for all these pieces of legislation, you know, at the end of the day it was her right, but you do then think, you know, the mental capacity act comes in. You know, what is capacity? You know, it's very clear when somebody is way out there, but when somebody appears to you as a very rational, sensitive human being and yet they're saying something to you that you think it's a bit difficult for you to understand, um, it gets tricky. (Community mental health occupational therapist)

In this example from study 3 a nurse consultant recognises a new situation: the home's *covert* medication *policy* being *in conflict with sectioning a patient*, and a new activity *managing in a different way*:

> One example of a case that I'm working with at the moment is a, is a lady who's in a, in a residential care home, who is non-compliant with some of her medication at times and the GP informed the home that the only way they could, um, supply the medicine in a covert manner was to have her sectioned. Well that's incorrect from two elements, one is that there's a covert medication policy anyway and the second is if the person is sectioned they can't remain in a residential home.
>
> So the staff all panicked saying 'Well, that means we'll have to get rid of her and we don't want to, she's been here three years and we love her to bits. And the daughter is in tears and we don't know what to say to her.' So it's, you know, saying to the GP 'We do need to manage it, but there is a different way.' While not offending his professional interpretation of what needs to happen, say to the daughter 'It's okay, we can work through this, but we need to have a case conference, etc.' And saying to the staff 'Well, what's happening here?' And then when I've reviewed the meds chart this lady is getting an inverted sleep pattern and she's actually missing meds because the meds are getting later and later in the day and she's not having regular medication, so then they're relying on PRM and it's just getting a complete mess. So we've sorted that bit out, but sometimes it's having the time to work with individuals and they often can come up with their own solutions. (Nurse consultant mental health)

From an interview with Sheila in study 5, here is another example of productive recontextualisation where Sheila thinks through her role as a nurse and states her role clearly in terms of her expectations of what she should achieve – challenge the trust to be *patient focused*:

> After a meeting with a big inner city NHS trust, I travel back to the CCG offices with Sheila and an administrator:

> Got bus back with Sheila and administrator who referred to tensions which Sheila said were around Hoare Frost trust being a typical medically led trust which wasn't that transparent and [that] Sheila's role was to push them to be transparent and patient focused. She gave example of the rise in A and E throughout which the trust saw in terms of a business model i.e. a good thing as they increased their income. She saw it from a patients' perspective 'it must be horrid being [in] a busier A and E' but when she challenged them over this, 'they don't get it'.

Tessa, like Sheila, draws on what she sees as a core nursing value in both her practice role and as a GBN: to be the patient voice and advocate:

> I think having, having your feet in practice, it's just so beneficial for patients. So you know how to negotiate, you know how to navigate the system and help them, and all that sort of thing, and that's the thing that I feel I'm really good at as well. And then this role enables me to make sure that that part, parts of their journey are as safe and as effective as we can possible make them.

A second GBN describes her emerging ability and confidence in putting knowledge to work in her role as a GBN after working for a primary care trust in an executive role. Primary care trusts (PCTs) were the precursor to clinical commissioning groups (CCGs). She describes her first thoughts about wanting to get involved in a different aspect of nursing: '*So, I thought that I would want, I wanted to get into, more around service redesign*', and her recognition that she didn't want to stop because by then she was enjoying the work: '*quite involved*' although it was '*exhausting*':

> So, I thought that I would want, I wanted to get into, more around service redesign, so I applied for the PCT nurse job, and got it, so that was in 2008 maybe. So I was on the PCT for a few years and then obviously when it became CCG I thought, I don't want to stop, so I'll carry on doing this sort thing. Because then it was, so I was quite involved in PCT, practice based commissioning, so, looking at exactly that, looking at pathways, looking at how we can redesign things, so when we came to the CCG obviously we were in shadow form, and then I got, I was allocated the quality and safety role. Which I've loved really, it was a major challenge to begin with and I kept thinking to myself, why, I don't even know why I'm putting myself under this stress, but it was just because there was just me and [my colleague], and it was incredibly stressful ... it's quite, it was incredibly time consuming, labour intensive, and exhausting ...

In another section of the interview she explains why she has stuck with this exhausting work: '*I think I use a different set of skills*'; and she goes on to explain how these skills have emerged in this GBN role:

There are some of them, that you use, so when we first started it was all, it was quite a, we had quite combative relationships with providers. They were used to being beaten with sticks by the PCT, about failing over healthcare acquired infections or whatever. Whereas me and [my colleague] came along and decided that actually we would work with them, with the providers to help them to be able to fix these problems. We haven't done it, but it's so, it was like squeezing blood out of a stone trying to get any information, particularly from some of the bigger providers over the road, and now, I wouldn't say we've got complete transparency but we have got, we get a huge amount more information because we see us actually trying to help them. And some of that is then coming back to GB and saying, they've not got enough money to be able to operate in this way. So if we then primed them a little bit to be able to work seven days a week on endoscopy or whatever, then actually, so they see us being, trying to help them, and so it's made the relationships more open, really. So they are quite different skills but they are, but transferable negotiation skills really.

Conclusions

These data seem to us to clearly illustrate WR: the healthcare professionals included in these data (nurses, occupational therapists and social workers) show that they theorise in practice in the face of huge organisational change. The acts of interpretation we've presented show that these experienced healthcare professionals are in the midst of role changes, service reorganisation and restructuring and at times, some of them are facing redundancy or their colleagues are. Their thinking and reflection serve to help them adjust to changes in their workplaces and offer examples of theorising in practice. Like the newly qualified nurses and the student nurses in Chapter 5, they theorise about their professional identity as they struggle to justify their:

- nursing roles and activities including extended roles
- purpose
- leadership.

Like the nurses in studies 1 and 2, a key feature of their theorising is the knowledge and their ability to learn and produce knowledge for their practice. They also show an impressive ability to manage ambiguity, complexity and conflict. Again, these data show how they:

- thought about the reasons why they care in particular ways
- articulated to each other in handovers or in case conferences the rationale of what the nursing care is based on
- thought through ethical practice.

While the fertility clinic appeared to have a well-organised and well-integrated learning and leadership model, the WR described in studies 3 and 5 seemed less reliant on workplace factors such as time and predictability, gradual release and enacted knowledge to support learning. Indeed, these healthcare professionals seemed not to think of themselves as lifelong learners engaged in continuous learning as part of their professional development nor do they describe support from management to assist them in their adjustment to new roles or reorganised teams and workplaces. Instead, these healthcare professionals seem remarkably resilient although they show evidence of stress. Their support seems to come from cohesive work teams and their ability to theorise in practice. In these respects, they demonstrate the capabilities and judgement of knowledgeable practitioners, able to read complex situations and act accordingly with professional interdependence and a degree of personal autonomy.

We now move on to discuss learner recontextualisation in Chapter 7.

7

Theorising in practice through learner recontextualisation

Chapter objectives

- Discuss learner recontextualisation (LR) and factors such as gradual release which may enhance LR
- Illustrate how learners make sense of learning–learner recontextualisation and thus theorise in practice drawing on data from the five studies described in Chapter 4
- Explore nurses' motivations for learning as well as related personal outcomes, and analyse the associations that are attached to different learning environments by employees

Introduction

In this chapter, we illustrate a second recontextualisation practice, learner recontextualisation – how nurses (again, no matter what stage of their career they may be) make sense of learning. Kersh et al. (2011a) argue that much of learning in work in advanced industrialised societies is predicated upon the ability and willingness of the individual worker (or nurse in our case) to engage with learning, to become a lifelong learner. Learning and acquiring skills through a range of experiences, including a learner's own life experiences, facilitate links and mutual interaction between learning, work and personal lives. Thus 'learners' spatial associations with their workplaces are often perceived as positive, as they may contrast with their previous negative experiences associated with formal education and training (e.g. schools or colleges)' (Kersh et al., 2011b: 3). In nursing, these spatial associations with workplaces as sites of learning are problematic as student nurses experience and/or perceive a split between university (theory) and practice. The ensuing and continuously reproduced theory–practice split sets up a tension between sites of learning. In this chapter we present data from all five studies described in Chapter 4 to illustrate learner recontextualisation, which shows learners theorising in practice as a way to integrate different forms of knowledge across different sites of learning.

Learner recontextualisation

This domain of putting knowledge to work describes ways in which learners make sense of learning contexts, the ways in which they creatively personalise their learning and thus develop professional identities. Learners draw on their prior disciplinary knowledge and on their prior and current work experiences in order to engage with the teaching, learning and assessment strategies and eventually their new work roles. These processes are facilitated when learners develop meta-cognitive strategies; and when learning partners work together to help the learners, whether students or newly qualified practitioners, to see connections and make sense of the whole process.

What learners make of these recontextualisation processes varies according to their personal characteristics and the scope for action that they have, individually and collectively, in work environments. Together with their prior learning and tacit knowledge, opportunities and affordances for learning may be unequally distributed (see Evans et al., 2004, 2006). However, these inequalities are not set for ever. Learner recontextualisation may take place through the strategies learners themselves use to bring together and put to work different forms of knowledge they have gained through the programme. Opportunities to engage with work, working with learning partners in college and workplaces and observing, enquiring and working with more experienced people in the workplace, may offer ways to redress inequalities.

These learner recontextualisation processes are part of a process through which nurses think and feel their way towards a sense of professional identity. The ways in which people forge identities, individually and collectively, within and through their practices are well captured by Kirpal and Simone (2004), who showed how professionals from contrasting fields (nursing and IT professionals) radiate different senses of themselves as particular kinds of workers as well as people with particular personal interests and commitments. These senses of self are thus multi-faceted, and represent the variety of ways in which people position themselves in relation to their employment, professional development and other purposeful activities in their lives (Drevdahl and Canales, 2020). For example, while Helen hasn't nursed anyone in hospital for over a decade, her professional identity and the knowledge she draws on in work and life mean she sees herself and explains herself to others through her identity as a nurse. Her self, if you like, can only be explained through her professional life as well as her personal life because the two are integrated. As roles change so too do facets of professional identity; for example when a frontline nurse moves into a supervisory role (or an educational and later research role as in Helen's case) shifts in their professional identity occur. The processes of thinking and feeling one's way into the enactment of new and changing roles are something that continues through working life and beyond it (as Helen has found). Holland et al.'s (1998) notion of figured worlds has offered a theory of self and identity that was used by Gill (2013) in understanding these formative experiences in the fragmented and constantly changing world of newcomers to clinical medical practice. Gill's research highlighted ways in which, where figured worlds are constantly changing, what one learns is how to vary performance, how to fit in, how to recontextualise forms of knowledge to make knowledge useful and how to 'keep a narrative of identity going over a constantly changing terrain' (2013: 123). Professional identity development also refers to new entrants coming to identify with others who participate in the same profession. For many workers, much of this development takes place within relatively stable work groups and overlapping social networks. However, an identity is not fashioned merely through enactment of practice. A strong degree of reflexivity is required as the worker starts to inhabit a role with identity at best only partly formed. The self-reflection to make the transition into the new identity entails both on reflection-in-action and on reflection after the event (Hinchcliffe, 2013: 52). This period of identity formation as a worker is a destabilising and potentially creative process which we have previously described as a liminal process where troublesome knowledge is processed to form new knowledge for work (Allan et al., 2015). In liminal learning spaces students and workers reformulate knowledge into new patterns. The process of liminality as a worker develops between different workplaces or across stages becomes transformative. While Cousin (2006) suggests that the learner enters the liminal state to engage with mastery of a project, learning in her model is affective and cognitive. Drawing on work by Hökkä et al. (2017), we suggest that learning is also social and embodied, developed through daily interactions. Students may be described as 'feeling' their way into a professional identity. This has been underplayed in the literature on threshold concepts and in Benner's theory of novice to expert (1984).

Professional learning might be interpreted as a way in which adults exercise *agency* in forging what they perceive, at any given time, to be their professional career paths or trajectories. Agency can be considered from the perspective of the processes that underpin the directing of action in the practices of their day-to-day work. In Emirbayer and Mische's (1998) temporal conception of agency, routines, habits and beliefs are brought from the past into the contingencies of the present moment, and agentic action reflects not only these habits, routines and beliefs *but also* the conceptions of the acting individual of what the possible outcomes, both proximal and distal, might be. Yet it is not just routines, habits and beliefs which are brought into the contingencies of the present moment but a variety of forms of knowledge, ranging from personal and tacit knowledge to the specialist scientific and professional forms of knowledge that fundamentally differentiate professional work. Knowledge is therefore 'put to work' in all forms of agentic action and is integral to an understanding of the social processes that not only characterise particular professions but also distinguish between them.

Agency is expressed in the processes of negotiation of the activities and relationships of professional practice, throughout working life. It is bounded in the negotiation of the organisationally and structurally embedded limits and the possibilities of the particular employment relationship. The reflexive processes of structuration involved in negotiating the requirements and expectations of a regulated profession in the NHS differ profoundly from the constant reinventions of the self that characterise the pursuit of agency work. Further sources of variation come from the input of practitioners themselves as they put knowledge to work, as well as from wider professional affordances and societal forces that tend to produce socially reproductive as well as potentially transformative learning. This interplay between professionals and their work/learning environment is illustrated in Helen's work into discriminatory practices towards overseas trained nurses' learning in the NHS (Allan, 2010; Allan et al., 2009a) (Box 7.1).

Contexts are not 'backdrops' for agency but constitutive of agency. The organisation, work team or individual can be taken as the point of departure. Furthermore, each individual's personal history can be considered a platform for their coming to know and making sense of what is encountered in workplaces and in their wider professional lives (Hökkä et al., 2017). This sense-making process both shapes and reflects the person's intentionality and agency in the ways in which they engage with work roles, as shown recently by Vähäsantanen et al. (2017). Analyses of how individuals engage with the affordances of work – what work offers them and can do for them – shows that the distribution of affordances is far from benign and is associated with the occupational hierarchies that operate with different degrees of visibility in organisations. See Box 7.1 for an illustration of these relationships.

Box 7.1   Agency and structuration in learning in the NHS: discriminatory practices in mentoring overseas nurses

The study: Valuing and Recognising the Talents of a Diverse Healthcare Workforce, undertaken by the University of Surrey, Open University and the Royal College of Nursing.

This work showed barriers to effective and non-discriminatory practice when mentoring overseas nurses within the NHS and the care home sector in the UK. Barriers included a lack of awareness about how cultural differences affect mentoring and learning for overseas nurses during their period of supervised practice prior to registration with the UK Nursing and Midwifery Council.

Data were collected using interviews undertaken with 93 overseas nurses, 24 national and 13 local managers and mentors from six research sites involving UK healthcare employers in the NHS and independent sectors in different

(Continued)

regions of the UK. The findings showed that overseas nurses are discriminated against in their learning by poor mentoring practices; equally, from these data, it appears that mentors are ill-equipped by existing mentor preparation programmes to mentor overseas-trained nurses from culturally diverse backgrounds. Recommendations are made for improving mentoring programmes to address mentors' ability to facilitate learning in a culturally diverse workplace and thereby improve overseas nurses' experiences of their supervised practice.

The authors argue in their report and subsequent papers that the agency expressed by overseas nurses as they negotiated their learning with mentors in the workplace was bounded and in many cases restricted by the organisationally and structurally embedded limits and possibilities of the particular employment relationship in the NHS. Ultimately, the interplay between the institutionally racist NHS with the informal racism of the UK workforce acted to disempower any agency overseas nurses used to learn effectively in the NHS.

The REOH report is available at: www.yumpu.com/en/document/view/8762599/valuing-and-recognising-the-talents-of-a-diverse-healthcare-rcn

Agentic practice

Learner recontextualisation refers to the processes whereby learners develop their professional and/or vocational expertise and identity and, in so doing, demonstrate an appreciation of their chosen occupation and their reasons for wanting to join it. The development of expertise and identity contributes significantly to sustaining their motivation to engage with the other processes of recontextualisation. Learners learn how to fit in and how to rework their knowledge to make it useful, while sustaining a narrative of their own personal professional development over time.

What learners make of the other recontextualisation domains or processes varies according to personal characteristics, the group/cohort of which they are part, the scope for action they have in any particular environment and the extent to which they exercise their own agency, and the nature of the learning activities they are asked to undertake. Self-generated recontextualisation strategies sometimes involve learners in:

- sharing 'war stories' with one another and their lecturers and, in the process, creating new understanding and insights about practice.

Learners sometimes have to be supported in the workplace to think and feel their way into their professional expertise and identity. This can take a number of forms:

- engaging in 'learning conversations' helps them to articulate more explicitly their growing understanding of practice and paves the way for them to write more critically-based assignments
- being stretched through opportunities to work at the next level and thereby providing learners with a more holistic grasp of the connections between aspects of practice (Hökkä et al., 2017).

Factors enhancing or working against learner recontextualisation processes

The same factors which enhance or work against work recontextualisation affect learner recontextualisation: time and predictability, gradual release, enacted new knowledge. When discussing learner recontextualisation, we must consider the individual abilities and strategies (personal, cognitive, emotional) as well as their social and cultural capital in navigating and negotiating their way through the learning environment (Allan, 2011; Allan et al., 2011).

Gradual release

Gradual release is deployed by practitioners in colleges and by workplace managers, supervisors and mentors to sequence the knowledge elements of their programme to develop learners' theoretical understanding alongside their skill development. It's a learning device to support learners to move from a college to a practice environment via the gradual iterative release of responsibility from teacher to learner; supervisor to learner; and mentor to learner. The gradual release of responsibility to the learner involves learners being given incremental opportunities across the axis of time and predictability.

Time and predictability

Learners strengthen their skill repertoires through extended exposure to tools and equipment with which they are already familiar. They learn by making mistakes in a controlled, closely supervised and sheltered environment, but one that progressively resembles the workplace itself. They move from predictable to more unpredictable tasks where some of the complexities of real-life work (and its artefacts) are built into the learning experience.

What learners make of these recontextualisation processes varies according to personal characteristics, their experience and the ways in which they express their individual agency, the features of their group or cohort and the scope for action they have in any particular environment. Learner recontextualisation takes place through the strategies learners themselves use to bring together knowledge gained through the programme and internalised from working with more experienced people in the workplace. Moreover, for full engagement to occur, learning has to be situated, and made sense of, in three ways: in practical activity; in the culture and context of the workplace learning environment; and in the socio-biographical features of the learner's life. Together with prior learning and tacit knowledge, these features are unequally distributed (Evans et al., 2004, 2006). The data we present in this chapter show how these strategies involve learners in the creation of new knowledge, insights and activities.

Enacted knowledge

The final activity which contributes to learner recontextualisation is enacted knowledge, which is achieved through working with others. Learners come to self-embody knowledge cognitively and practically. They can use knowledge as a set of resources to develop professional and academic identity together, using both curriculum and workplace knowledge as 'test-benches'. A testing approach extends beyond application of general principles. It entails active noticing – being alert to what makes situations similar and what makes them different and requiring a different response. It also entails observing and learning from the experiences of others; enquiring into and reflecting upon the situations of challenges that experienced practitioners have faced and resolved. Thinking and feeling one's way into a professional identity is facilitated by such practices as engaging in 'learning conversations' and hearing 'war stories'; articulating developing understandings to others; asking questions purposefully and being stretched through opportunities to work at the next level. Engaging with role models, with critical insights into what it is of value they are modelling, is also part of this process of thinking and feeling one's way into a professional identity.

As in Chapters 5 and 6, we now illustrate our theory with data from the five research studies we introduced in Chapter 4.

Illustrations of learner recontextualisation in clinical practice

LR depends on an individual learner's ability and willingness to engage with learning, to become a lifelong learner. Being a lifelong learner allows someone to learn and acquire skills through a range of experiences including their own life experiences and to facilitate links and mutual interaction between learning, work and leisure. Such an individual will show an ability to make sense of learning contexts, and be creative in the ways in which they personalise their learning and thus develop a professional identity. The extract in Box 7.2 demonstrates an act of interpretation from an interview with an NQN in study 2 who had focused mainly on her difficulties with working with HCAs. At the end of the interview she described her awareness of how her learning had changed in an individual act of interpretation which illustrates learning recontextualisation.

Box 7.2   Reflection leading to learner recontextualisation

How can I, say with me, umm, I used to be shy, very shy, and then, [laughs] exactly, and then all of a sudden, one day, I think I came to this hospital, I just thought 'do you know what, I've got to get over this', because I'm not going to get anywhere, like I wasn't standing up, not standing up, but I wasn't standing up for myself, I was sort of a little shadow, I used to sort of think I'll just get on with it and just not approach anybody, but now, I've decided. All of a sudden I felt ... Yeah, hmm, yeah I think because as a student I didn't, I didn't, my academic side of things was a bit, not poor,

> but I wasn't an A star student, I was a C, you know, I was always 'just' passing my assignments and some of them I failed and I had to re-take so my confidence was always being knocked back and knocked back, now I had to learn, to speak, I'm going to get there one day, I will get there, I'm determined, and then I did, and I thought 'well if I can get through the assignments that are killing me, absolutely killing me, then I can, I can ask someone to do a blood pressure for me, and I can approach my Sister when I've got a problem'.

The key moment of LR, where she sees the whole picture and brings together her thoughts and feelings about her abilities, her agency, her social capital and her sense of identity as an NQN, comes as she says: '*all of a sudden I felt …*' and then again in the phrase: '*I had to learn, had to speak*'. After describing her hesitancy and shyness, she repeats in the end *I can* and finishes by saying *I can* again. And just before the end of the interview, she reiterates this point of recontextualisation where she articulates a personal learning strategy:

> No, I just felt I'm not going to get anywhere here if I keep doing this, I've got to stand up for myself, I've got to talk to people, it has helped.

There were many examples of nurses having moments of clarity where they described understanding their feelings about their role and the learning that is required.

> Yeah, just from time and experience and maybe it's like you don't prioritise one thing one time and then you just look back on it and think 'I should have done that first …'

> Yeah, and then I can always look back and think 'oh yeah, I still need to do that', but I just hold it all in my head, I remember and sort of go through it and then you're like I've done that now I need to do this.

In comparing data from all five studies, we argue that LR is contingent upon context in complex ways. In study 4 particularly, it appeared that the context of infertility and working intimately with couples, and the shared gendered experience with female patients, shaped the development of LR. In the extract below is a description of LR arising from the personal and intimate nature of the work with infertile couples:

> … um, I think just generally having experience of being female, although I haven't got children, you know the delight and joy that babies bring to a lot of people and therefore being at the other end of things people who can't have children, From my point of view a field that would be very difficult to come in as a young inexperienced nurse. I think a new qualified nurse would find it quite difficult.

Probably like many nurses facing new roles, fertility nurses described LR in their struggle with the process and consequences for themselves and their patients of their extended specialist roles. Their theorising is revealed in their ability to make connections and see the whole of the context in which they care, their sense of agency and professional identity. This is captured in the following extract in an act of interpretation when describing a general openness to a patient's or couple's emotional wellbeing:

> I think we're better than doctors at picking up certain signs, non-verbal communication, we're trained to look at the way people communicate [with] each other. We're not trained to just give information to people, we're trained to listen. And I think a lot of doctors are trained to just come in, do their bit, give information to the patient, decide what they're going to do and then they're out. While we are interpreting how the patient's handled that information, what impact it's had on them ... you see, they come for their first visit and I know you shouldn't be assessing their relationship for stability but if one of them spends all the time looking out the window, you immediately know there's not something not quite right. And it might take several visits before you find out what it is, but once you pick something like that up, you slow things down, and try to give them time and space and that's coming from non-verbal communication and looking at them and really seeing them.

Complexity of learner recontextualisation

As in WR, LR involves a complex dynamic within teams and within defined workplaces. While LR involves personal learning and growing confidence and agency, it also requires the NQN to see the whole team's needs and see the connections between their position vis-a-vis those they manage daily. In this data extract, the HCA describes the dynamics as an NQN struggles to work in a team with HCAs and '*power goes to their head*'. It reinforces for her that for LR to take place, the whole situation at work needs to be understood and integrated into an NQN's practice.

> Being a healthcare assistant makes a good nurse because they understand, they understand what the ward's like, they understand anyway how to respect us healthcare's you know, and they don't take us for granted which I personally find is when they come straight in from Uni, come straight onto the ward, the power really goes to their head and it's like 'oh I can tell this person what to do' and that starts us being a bit reluctant to go to them kind of thing so, and that's what I personally find.

However, NQNs described complex relationships with HCAs which were frequently poor or difficult to negotiate. These relationships added another layer of complexity to LR. This NQN describes this complexity and her feeling that she's not respected by an HCA:

> Mmm, you sort of feel ... yeah, it's annoying because you know your jobs you need to get done, but if they've said that they're going to do this and that first and they're not willing to come and help you, then that makes you feel like they're not working with you as a team. And that they don't respect your position and they don't feel that you know what you're doing, it sort of feels like that and then you start feeling like you're a bad nurse and stuff.

LR is complex therefore and can take time. This ability to accomplish LR was described by participants across the studies as *seeing the whole*.

Seeing the whole in LR

Seeing the whole is an important feature of LR and shows an awareness of the interplay between the context of work, individual and repeated situations at work and one's own positioning within the whole (the workplace as a whole). Box 7.3 exemplifies 'seeing the whole' for an NQN. In this data extract, an NQN describes the interplay between his own agency and actions, '*his authority*', and the workplace as a whole, which he refers to as '*level in the ward team*'.

Box 7.3 Seeing the whole in practice

Yeah, I don't think it [delegation] was something that I was initially very good at but I think it's something I'm picking up now as I've kind of got used to it within my kind of new role, do you know what I mean, because as I say before this as a student I didn't really have that chance because you don't really, you haven't got the – not authority, but the level in the ward team [? ward hierarchy] to be able to kind of hand out tasks as much I think as a student nurse.

And he goes on to describe how he recontextualises and sees the whole, '*just order it in your head*':

There's all kinds of, because there's so many different facts that go into each different decision like number one for like a medication, patients having ... that medication must be given on time so that one must be [slaps paper] done at certain times and there's, then there's things that can wait and you do, you just order it in your head don't you?

His final phrase, '*you just order it in your head don't you?*', summarises the complexity of recontextualisation – it feels like it's done in his head but has temporal ('*taken so long*') and contextual ('*working with a student*') elements, as he goes on to describe:

Yeah, that's why it's taken so long, because I do, do that and especially with, [when] I am working with a student nurse as well.

In this interview, another NQN makes an explicit reference to integrating learning in university and learning in practice to create a fuller or whole understanding of his practice:

Like we did a module about team roles at work, that helps me a lot in delegation. And also the idea of working as a team as in ... making someone think that, making someone, showing someone that we're working together and not, we're not against each other if you know what I mean ... So, that, I learnt from that module, team roles at work and Uni, I tried to remember the examples that the lecturers used to give us, yeah, and now I look, I look back and I say yeah, I now know what you were talking about kind of thing.

In study 3, there were a number of detailed descriptions of LR which rely on sustained personal reflection on spatial associations between sites of learning. This is possibly because the healthcare professionals (HCPs) we interviewed were working repeatedly with patients in the community with long-term conditions and often knew them very well. There were therefore opportunities for reflection on learning as part of practice created from repeated exposure to the same patients which were not available for NQNs in a more quickly paced acute care setting. Acts of interpretation in study 3 were not always described as acts involving seperate activities but rather as a sense of relationships which developed over time; often through articulating an underlying approach or philosophy of care to approaching patients and their families. An example is given in Box 7.4. In this extract, the health visitor describes her awareness of her new situation as a heath visitor where her professional practice is substantially and philosophically different to her practice as a nurse. She recognises that her new field of practice requires a response and uses knowledge – theoretical, procedural and tacit – in acts of interpretation in an attempt to bring the activity, its setting and its underlying values under conscious control.

Box 7.4   LR developing over time in long-term health visiting practice

It can be because I think the thing I found when I first qualified, because when you're a staff nurse you're working at a level where you are, um, I mean obviously huge skills and, but much more about helping the family, not, you do use assessment skills, because that's what nurses do, but you're assessing at a different level and one thing I found the most steep learning curve to do my degree and to do my qualification was that actually you can't always help everybody. As a nurse that's what you want to do, that's why you go into the profession. Even if you're helping somebody to die, you're trying to help them have a dignified death, but with this it's much more complex than that and there are times when, you know, another domestic violence call has come in and you think 'Oh.' You just really want to help this woman, but actually there's only so much you can do and I think that can be extremely frustrating, but you do learn over time that you have to kind of let that go and that you can't solve everybody's problems.

The same health visitor gave another example later in the interview to show how thinking in and on practice helps her to bring professional practice under her conscious control:

I do get frustrated and sometimes I just think 'Why am I doing this?' Um, and then you go and do a visit and you realise you have made a difference to somebody or you do, it sounds really awful, but you do a nice normal visit, you have a nice little family with nice little children and everything is going well for them and you think 'Oh, there is somebody out there with everything.' Because I think the danger of doing always the difficult families is that you, and it's probably the same for Social Services, you forget that there is a nice, um, normal, for want of a better word, side to your job as well, but the way it is, is that we do get embroiled in all these quite difficult and complex families and things, so.

Another act of interpretation from study 3 illustrates *seeing the whole*. It involves an occupational therapist reflecting on how policy, creating '*prompt access to psychological therapies in primary care*', may change occupational therapists' roles by emphasising one aspect of their underpinning knowledge base rather than another:

And of course the new ways of working now, I think there's a risk there, although I understand, you know, that the kind of the broad philosophy I think is a good one in terms of having prompt access to psychological therapies in primary care, I have a slight concern that what's happening here is that, um, those of us, the few remaining OTs, that people have their sights set on us is that we'll deliver the agenda and it will be all psychological, but [they] forget that OT isn't just a psychological treatment. Um, you know, we use aspects of psychology and, you know, as part of what we do, but there's also a whole other, um, framework which comes from theories around, you know, occupation and meaning ... So I am concerned that we could be highjacked to be delivering in ... management groups when actually we actually need to be attacking the core of why people aren't able to engage with activities that bring meaning into their life.

This occupational therapist returned to this theme of the knowledge and thus the practice base of professional occupational therapy practice being threatened later in the interview, as she describes trying to retain philosophy of care or values from professional occupational practice:

I try my hardest, often at the detriment of the other things I'm supposed to do like filling in contact sheets and I'm always in trouble, um, but I think [pause] I don't know, I think I probably have enough time to maybe ... I don't feel that I have enough time to do the treatment interventions that I would want to because often practical things take a long time, you know, so if you're going to support someone to cook a meal and you need to shop for it it's going to take, you know, a couple of hours maybe and yet, you know, we're supposed to have, you know, fifty minute slots and ten minutes to write your notes and on to the next one. Um, and similarly, you know, any kind of skills building you have to maybe do that over a period of time and we've been accused of seeing people for too long and spending too much time with them, which I thought 'Well, that's interesting, I've not been accused of that before.'

And finally, she says she feels like a '*dinosaur*', threatened with extinction in the face of service reorganisation and policy where professional knowledge is organised out of a new system:

It feels like we're kind of it's hanging in the balance and it could go either way. There are some people who believe it's already gone and they're setting their sights on sort of retraining as psychological therapists, um, and there are others who believe that it's quite important and so are fighting on. Maybe, you know ... dinosaur.

This sense of services being restructured to remove some forms of professional practice was also experienced by one of the nurse consultants we interviewed. However this district nurse consultant appears to feel more hopeful and has certainly acted to manoeuvre successfully through threats to her professional autonomy, in an example of learner recontextualisation:

Int: And then you said intermediate care has disappeared?

It's still there and, and the philosophy is still there in so much as we've got integrated teams, um, with a rehabilitation focus, but unfortunately the intermediate care was defined by, um, the Department of Health as being a, you know, limited amount of time the service would be offered and that was around about the six week mark and of course we realised that people might need longer than that. So what we're trying to do is actually design our services around the individual rather than actually make people fit into boxes and criteria, um, so we were really mindful of that. And, unfortunately, even with the flexibility of a joint service, there are still elements where people actually need to meet criteria in order to be accepted and I think that is actually changing the hearts and minds of the people working with the particular silos of the, of the services. And fortunately for me, because of my, um, role, I can move up and down and across all parts of the services, including the hospital and it does actually enable you, I hate the term, but the helicopter view, and it does enable you to see, um, all the trains where they are at the time and, um, and so you can actually you do get that overview and perhaps see where, where bits of the service or the referral pathways are a bit clunky and you can actually work with teams to actually help smooth those out.

Later in the interview she describes another example of successful networking and manoeuvring through a changed system to pursue her vision of care based on her knowledge and skills. She recognises a new situation, '*managing the back door to the community hospital*', as requiring a response and uses knowledge – theoretical, procedural and tacit – in acts of interpretation, '*being co-chair on a committee, in-reach into the hospital, wider view of what's happening'*, in an attempt to bring the activity and its setting under conscious control:

> I've been working with the local acute hospital, um, and I've been asked to co-chair as part of their overarching urgent care work on discharge planning and rehabilitation models. And as part of that work I've actually done more in-reach into the acute, um, hospital and also I now sit on the team meetings, the interdisciplinary team meetings at our community hospital. And again, that's enabled me to have this sort of wider view of what's happening in parts of the service and, as part of that, an outcome from that, I've now got all parts of our service to rotate into the weekly meetings at the community hospital. Because what I was finding was they were managing the front door of the hospital very well because the referral pathways in were clear, but the back door wasn't being managed so well and that's probably what we criticise our acute doing and we were doing exactly the same. So by drawing in other members of the team, like community nursing, like promoting independency, like rapid response, like domiciliary physio, is enabling those team members to influence the exit strategy, if you like, of the community hospital. And that's actually been, you know, quite valuable and it's helped the networking as well.

What strikes us about these two different extracts from the occupational therapist and the district nurse consultant, is the importance of identity as an attribute of learner recontextualisation which enables theorising in practice. The occupational therapist describes a Hobson's Choice of either failing to maintain a professionally distinct identity and professional practice or some kind of resistance work to maintain individual practice. And the nurse expressed confidence in her nursing voice in her descriptions of working with other professionals to make the reorganised system work for her patients.

However, seeing the whole may be an uncomfortable experience as these lecturers and practice educators acknowledge in a focus group interview in study 1. The lecturer feels that mentors aren't educated to teach following cuts to the traditional teaching and learning module mentors had to study until the early 2000s. As she says:

> My concerns with our mentorship programme is that it was pared to the bones for economic reasons and what was the old 998 which was about teaching has been lost. We now have to focus on documentation. That's an enormous part of the mentorship course and all the stuff about educational audit, the environment, and the bit about the theory of mentoring but there's very little time in that five days to … really discuss and to get to grips with one-to-one teaching.

In the same focus group, it was suggested that the ward culture could influence an orientation to teaching or not, as this practice educator says:

> I've heard some of my team say 'Oh, why have you done that?' 'Oh, because XX has told us to'. No actually we always explain the rationale for why we do that. But it's easier for people to say 'Oh because we do'. And there's very much a culture within our workforce which does that. A lot of our workforce are not doing [explaining] and our students aren't being brought up with that either.

How time and predictability, gradual release and knowledge enactment shape learner recontextualisation processes

We have argued in Chapters 5 and 6 that learning is mediated by three factors that recur in our explorations of the conditions and experiences that are associated with different modes of recontextualisation. These same three factors also shape learner recontextualisation.

Time and predictability

What is noticeable about our data in study 2 is that the NQNs working in busy wards are not (always) exposed to activities safely as a learner or through repeated exposure to the same predictable and repeated activity over time. In other professional fields where training is carried out in simulated environments, trainees are exposed step-by-step to greater levels of unpredictability under gradually increasing time pressures until they reach the point of being able to operate safely and effectively at the levels expected in a busy operating environment. In the example from a busy NHS ward (Box 7.5), the activity of giving intravenous antibiotics was threatened by the unpredictability of other events which interfered with the NQN's ability to give the prescribed antibiotics. The mistake which was made was not entirely within her control and serves to illustrate how the unpredictable nature of work in busy NHS wards may be a barrier to learning and attaining competency and fluency in activities. Ironically though, an additional factor which shapes recontextualisation may be learning through mistakes. In the example, the NQN describes how she has learnt to say no based on her learning from experience in order to avoid making mistakes which could have serious implications for her registration. As she says, the act of interpretation is revealed in her '*being aware of things that could happen*'.

Box 7.5   Time and predictability in learner recontextualisation

I was doing my medications in the bay and then we were short-staffed and the nurses in bay one … I was in bay three, and the nurses in bay one had to do the medication for bay one and bay four, because there wasn't a nurse in bay four, we were all sort of looking after bay four. And she just happened to go past and it was getting on for time, because we were short-staffed, and it was a very busy day, we had lots of discharges and new admissions and she said 'Would you mind helping me do the drugs for bay four?' and when I said 'Yeah, of course I will' … because I felt I had to help because we were short-staffed, and I had one IV to do, one IV antibiotic to do, so I basically took the drug with me into bay four, helped her do some of the medications in bay four, then I was going to do the IV antibiotic straightaway afterwards. But there was a fall from one of my patients in the toilet where the healthcare assistant was helping him to the toilet and he fell, [?? 0:25:05] ring the call bell afterwards, he tried to get [?? 0:25:07] and so I had to go away and sort that out. And then, by the time I came back to that IV antibiotic, it was already eight o'clock and that was when the night staff were coming in and, basically, they complained because it should have been given. But then it was my fault, but I was helping other people because we were short-staffed, so being short-staffed, then mucked up sort of my shifts and almost got me in trouble as well. So there's sort of a blame culture, you feel like you're doing the right thing at the time, then it can easily stab you in the back as well, so yeah, I could have had an incident form done on me then, but …

… it didn't happen …

… no, we did the antibiotic together and then when we got back down … because it should have been done, really, between six and seven and it was an hour out, but we managed …

Yeah, was this early on when you'd started?

No, this was just even a couple of weeks ago.

Oh, so would you call this one of your 'learning by mistakes'?

Yeah, because next time, I will just … it sounds really bad, I'm not going to help next time if I … I will get my jobs done first, maybe, get my important jobs done first rather than go and help someone.

Yeah, it must be tricky, yeah.

Yeah, because it was so short-staffed and I thought she's got two bays of drugs to do, and I wasn't planning on having that patient falling …

Of course not.

… and if that patient hadn't have fell, I would have got the antibiotic done on time, so yeah, it's just being aware of things that could happen.

In a quote from study 1, a 3rd year student describes time and predictability being used to ease the senior student into their transition to NQN. He explained that it wasn't easy to gain experience because of safety reasons, unlike when his uncle trained as a nurse:

My uncle says in his second year he was in charge of wards and was responsible. But it had to change. You have to be accountable for safe care and you can't just do things to patients. But we've been out of practice for a year during our second year and it felt very strange coming back [to a general ward].

This student recognised that being safe and accountable had left him feeling deskilled and he felt that on the mixed surgical ward they were given appropriate responsibility as 3rd years and expected to work as part of the team. Here, as 3rd year students, they were treated preferentially and their mentors allowed them to check intravenous (IV) drugs, run through IV lines, change IV lines all under supervision. And they appreciated that, as they would have to do those tasks when qualified, they wanted them *'under their belt'* before then.

In study 4, nurses were learning intricate and highly complex skills such as egg and sperm retrieval and embryo transfer (during IVF treatments). In this extract, the lead nurse describes how the unit has developed an interdisciplinary training protocol for ultra sound scanning among other procedures which all staff have to undertake. It involved repeating activities, having a mentor, being assessed and repeating a skill until the assessor is satisfied you are competent. This approach of repeat exposure over time and demonstration of predictable competence facilitates putting knowledge to work because to develop dexterity, practice is required:

You also have a role teaching doctors in their new role in the unit?

Yes assessing their scanning ability. Basically, if they have a problem with me assessing them, they take it to [consultant] because I have a responsibility to my patients in my care and the unit and I won't allow anybody unsafe to operate without saying something to them. So they have to take it really I'm afraid! I wouldn't allow them [to] operate without being safe on myself, so why should I allow them to do it unsafely on a patient? I think doctors are trained differently, see one, do one teach one and we have gone to great lengths to develop these protocols and say that you have to do this training and do a number of scans before you can do egg collections and to be supervised and why should it be any different for doctors. They may have the academic knowledge but academic knowledge isn't necessarily related to dexterity ...

She goes on to say that dexterity isn't enough for understanding at a deeper level, when learning to assess which treatment or investigation is needed for which couple:

... anybody can be trained to do procedures, egg collections, and that's not the critical thing. The critical thing is understanding what you're doing. And that only comes with time by seeing different scenarios by you have to use your brain every day, you can't go onto autopilot, you have to think about what you're doing, that's what makes it enjoyable for me. Because no two individuals are the same, no two couples are the same. Okay, a lot of the treatments are standard but you have to assess whether that standard treatment's suitable for that particular couple in front of you. That's part of the enjoyment of the job.

Gradual release

In the following extract, a WM appears to criticise NQNs' lack of confidence – *'they ask a lot of questions'* – instead of understanding that this *constant* questioning is a process of learning to gradually become confident to act on their own initiative:

Nowadays they seem to rely a lot on senior staff and they ask a lot of questions which is fine but I think sometimes they need to be a little bit ... to have some autonomy and think for themselves and, and do stuff individually rather than constantly, constantly ask, for my point of view I feel much more confident when I know things and I can do them on my own rather than having to ask my manager so I think I'm looking from the perspective from their perspective if you like because it must be hard constantly to have to rely on someone ...

She goes on to question whether they lack knowledge, courage or confidence as they don't seem to want to *do* it. She seems to imply that a gradual approach to learning is a crutch which prevents NQNs from becoming full professionals – '*it's like a button you know, telling them this is right*':

... so I don't know why, are they lacking on, on knowledge, where is that courage to be independent and take decisions in what they do ... they lacking confidence if you like, not necessarily knowledge, if you do question the student, the newly qualified nurses they did have the knowledge it's just that, it's like a button you know, telling them this is right, yeah, you can do this, you don't need to ask, what you're thinking is just right, just do it.

And a little later she acknowledges that NQNs do have knowledge but their questioning prevents them doing the job and becoming confident. She understands that she has put knowledge to work or recontextualised knowledge when she says, '*knowledge comes with practice*':

... because knowledge comes with practice most of the time and if you do work with, with nurses closely they do, we do have cases and everyday practice where they do come brilliant nurses and a lot of things comes to practice and it happens to me in the past you know, the more you, I've been on maternity leave recently, I came back, I panicked I thought I'd lost all my knowledge, so every, I do believe that everything comes with practice.

A questioning approach is generally regarded as a positive element in knowledge recontextualisation, when it is 'enquiring' in nature. But the quality and context of the questioning is also important. When a learner asks questions to elicit insights and explanations from practitioners whom the learner regards as knowledgeable, it is not necessarily an indicator of dependence and lack of confidence; it can signal the opposite. Such an enquiring approach supports learner recontextualisation; it helps in working things out. Mentors need to be able to facilitate learning both through understanding the question and its context, tolerating the question in the context and responding to answer the question.

However, as we've emphasised, learning isn't always possible in the clinical workplace; neither is gradual release. There seems to be a belief that gradual release isn't desirable for learning as a nurse. As the following quote from a nursing lecturer suggests, gradual release isn't possible because learning can only be achieved through doing; some aspects of being an NQN don't make sense or are not even recognised until the learner moves from senior student to NQN:

Yeah, yeah, it, sometimes it didn't, it didn't make sense, you know when you're a student and you're on the ward as a student some of these things we don't notice, you don't actually notice until you've become the person who needs to be doing it and I notice that, because as a student there's a lot, there's a lot I, I didn't really think that nurses had to go through until I became [an NQN].

Again, here an NQN saying that while she learnt at university and had experience, once she had her job as an NQN, '*actually, since I've had my job*', along with '*the fast pace*' and learning '*through mistakes*', she's been able to learn an '*awful lot*':

I got a lot of my experience at university, but I have to say, I've learnt an awful lot in the last eight months, actually, since I've had my job, because it's such a fast-paced ward, I've had to learn to keep up properly and you develop your role when you've qualified, I think, more than when you were unqualified because you have to just get on with it. And you learn through mistakes as well that you've made, and you learn to time-priority because when you're in charge of your bay, you may be a bit slow in the first couple of weeks, then you learn what you need to do properly.

Implicitly here she's acknowledging the learning at university but emphasising that even more learning has taken place in placement as a staff nurse, i.e. on qualifying, and gradual release has not been a big feature of her learning after qualifying.

Enacted knowledge

In study 4, the following example of a positive learning experience and environment was given by a fertility nurse. As well as describing enacted knowledge in learning conversations, she also describes gradual release facilitated by time and predictability:

I think it took approximately, everything was little bits by bits, after I did so many of one thing then I could do it on my own if I felt comfortable, um there's still lots of areas where I don't feel comfortable such as scanning, but everyone's really good and they'll come in.

Yeah, so you just call on people when you need extra support?

Yeah, and every once in a while I'll meet with [manager] and go through with how I think I'm doing and what she's noticed, if I've improved or if I still need to work on certain areas, quite regularly.

There were many examples of learning conversations between students and mentors and between peers where knowledge was clearly enacted and possible because of good interpersonal relationships. As in the observations of relationships between students and mentors from study 1:

Just last week I was stopped by a student in the corridor just to let me know how wonderful she thought her mentor had been. They had worked together closely in what the student described as a 'partnership' and she had been encouraged and supported by the mentor 'to do a lot of things.' She described it to me as 'a turning point' in her training. (Acute medicine morning shift)

Although I'm supernumerary, I'm kept very busy. I don't feel unsafe just very busy. Brenda's always around [the student's mentor]. (Day surgery morning shift)

I came onto the ward and the staff nurse and student (2nd year) are arranging shifts to work together. Staff nurse walked off from the station saying for the student to follow her which she didn't immediately. Staff nurse gestured 'come on' like there was a lead tying the student to her. They both laughed. (Day surgery late shift)

While the last extract may seem patronising, this mentor explained later to the researcher that ensuring students felt safe but at the same time gained competencies and confidence was very important to her. As she said,

I was a P2K [Project 2000] student and I'm sick of people saying 'P2K can't organize xyz'. One person actually said that 'P2K nurses, if there wasn't a tape measure, wouldn't fit TED stockings; they aren't flexible!' I had to say 'I'm sorry, I don't think so!' I promised myself I wouldn't let students go through what I went through.

There were also examples of barriers to enacted knowledge (Box 7.6). Barriers to enacted knowledge and therefore LR were described in study 1 predominantly as students feeling a lack of support and the opportunity for learning. Here students express their anger to Helen about a lack of any sort of relationship with mentors and other staff.

Box 7.6   Barriers to enacted knowledge in clinical workplace

Three 3rd year students complained of feeling left out and agreed that they 'feel students are seen as stupid, clumsy, and that we'll make mistakes'. One student added 'I resent this' (Emergency unit and surgery).

At coffee, student described how she felt they were told to be assertive and self-empowered in college and to be agents of change yet the NHS and nursing was hierarchical and bullying and she said 'I feel like I'm in the playground again. On ICU, nobody said goodbye to me when I left, too busy doing internet shopping, obsessing about off duty and character assassination of anyone coming into the unit.' She felt that staff referred to the students as 'the student' and staff didn't bother to learn their names; rarely felt part of the team. She used the word 'burden' to describe the mentoring relationship in the clinical areas (Day surgery morning shift; 3rd year, older, female, part-time student).

But barriers can also arise from the context of the clinical workplace; it's intimidating, stressful and confusing for newcomers. The mentor's role is to

(Continued)

> support the student to overcome these barriers and enacted conversations can be a way to do this:
>
> A lot of students when they come into [operating] theatre act like wall flowers and you can't really blame them because it is totally different to what they've seen. They will come in looking very uncertain, very unsure of literally where they stand, where they go and what they do and they seem to fall into two categories, the ones who push themselves forward and the ones who won't and the ones who push themselves forward I'm not too bothered about, it's the ones that are reluctant. Is it because they have never seen an operation before and it's a little bit unusual for them, or is it just because of the environment, or is it because nobody's spoken to them and why? So it's making them, for me, making them feel at ease and understanding what we're doing and why, that takes a bit of one on one discussion or finding themselves somebody who's able to talk to them so that they feel more at ease.

Iterations of time and predictability, gradual release and knowledge enactment potentially move the learner from interpretation to adaptive recontextualisation and then productive recontextualisation. The factors that facilitate and impede this process point to some optimal conditions for successful LR.

Adaptive recontextualisation

Successful LR includes an individual learner having an active learning attitude. The following extract from an NQN shows an active learning attitude as she describes consciously observing a more experienced nurse in order to learn. She then reflects on her learning from another setting and is able to create new knowledge or understanding to inform her current practice:

> I was in once with a lady who was my patient and she'd just been told that she had terminal bowel cancer and the bowel specialist nurses in there and they had a consultant in, so I went in as well, but I was watching how, I was using it, because I didn't, I didn't say anything because you know, I was watching it, how they dealt with, and I picked up a lot of really good communication skills from, from them. But also on the preceptorship, they taught us something called 'Sage and Thyme', I don't know if you're aware of that? ... It's fantastic, and, it was the palliative care nurses that did it and it was, erm, it all stands for something [bleep goes off], I've got the little card in my wallet that I can show you, and it's basically like putting yourself in the situation and then I can't remember what all they stand for [bleep goes off], but it's about, its, it's about protecting you, but protecting the patients, so it's getting straight to the point, no like waffle, get you straight by saying, [bleep goes off], 'you look upset, what can I do', and it's about, erm, asking them who they have to help them, what you can do for them and then breaking

off, and not getting you know [bleep goes off] involved too much and not spending lots of, getting to the point and helping a patient but without spending too much time. (Sage and Thyme: www.sageandthymetraining.org.uk/)

And from study 3, a health visitor describes a way of thinking which allows her to learn and adapt through acts of interpretation:

Oh, hugely, yes, hugely because, um, I get quite, I enjoy looking at ways of doing things differently and not just doing things because we've always done them that way and perhaps sometimes it's irritating to other people, but I think we have to look at why we're doing things sometimes. I mean that's the whole idea of having generations of new trainees is to keep everything fresh and that's what some of the, the governance and particularly things like the NICE guidelines have to look at and 'Why are things being done that way? How can we improve them?' And making sure that we're all doing it in a certain way. Because it's very easy to get comfortable and do things a certain way because that's how it's always been done. Um, when you've trained more recently you have to look into the research on why it's been done, not just because. It's a totally different way of learning, isn't it?

Despite the complexity and burden of adapting to new processes, nurses in study 3 described adaptive recontextualisation:

... we would aim to be spending 45–60 minutes with patients on a visit, unless it's giving medicines or unless they are saying, 'I don't want you here for an hour, it's my evening, thanks very much.' I think patients get much more time with us than they would if they were on the ward for instance. (Community psychiatric nurse)

... so I mean, certainly the actual factual feedback we have from the patients is that they prefer the service as it now. They much prefer having treatment, being treated in their own homes as opposed to hospital care, so I think it's had a massive impact. (Community nurse mental health)

For one nurse manager, adaptive recontextualisation was described as she thought about how she was helping her staff to adapt to change:

If you want people to work together, get them to talk to each other. It's probably saying really things will be better – putting names to faces and all of that kind of self-system stuff works very well. (Senior mental health nurse)

In this extract, the experienced nurse consultant describes using acts of interpretation on a regular basis to manage similar activities in new settings:

And I think the other thing is I'm able to, because of my experiences right from before I trained, I worked as a care worker through to a nurse consultant, therefore I'm able to adjust the information and the knowledge base I'm giving to people to their level without being condescending. So, and that's been very helpful in working with the residential homes in managing people with delirium, especially, and dementia because, as you know, people with dementia are eight times more susceptible to developing the delirium they bounce into hospital, they get admitted because they're quite fragile, they then get a hospital acquired infection and then, you know, it's massive ... and then you're heading towards a nursing home. So just enabling staff to feel in control and knowing what they're doing by providing them with simple information and support just to manage them through, you know, saying 'You just need to get them through the first seventy-two hours, we might have to add extra medicine to enable you to do that, but if we add that then this increases this risk. So if you give them more medicine it means that might increase their risk of fall, their tissue viabilities, we need to do this as well.' And we monitor it on a daily basis and people who we've previously, not we, but who have previously bounced through the system several times, we've had quite a good success rate in keeping them where they are. (Nurse consultant mental health)

Adaptive recontextualisation comes from immersion in a field of practice where the learner is reflexively engaging in activities in new situations which stimulate her or him to think through existing knowledge and adapt it to familiar situations. In the following data extract, the fertility nurse describes how this is achieved:

These are areas where we are specialized in and we have more knowledge in this area, this small area, than a lot of doctors have, and more than any doctor will ever have unless they work in the field full time. So I think although [it] isn't a formal training, we're exposed to the knowledge and the field every day of our practice.

Productive recontextualisation

The examples from study 4 show how the nurses we interviewed about their extended specialist roles were able to change the activity or its context in an attempt to respond to a new situation and produce new knowledge about their practice and that of their colleagues – productive recontextualisation. These nurses described learning to be aware of feelings in patient interactions. This psychodynamic approach to working with feelings is fairly well documented in fertility and women's health nursing more widely (Allan, 2011a). In the following extract the nurse describes using her feelings in the patient encounter to assess and manage difficult situations such as pregnancy loss:

You've a little bit of a hint anyway from what they're telling you. They'll have had some bleeding, a little discomfort and you tend to get an inkling and they themselves will know and they'll say 'Oh Eliza, I don't think it's going to be there'.

And again in the following quote, the nurse compares her extended specialist role in which she's allowed to use her feelings and be with the patients with sonographers, who were not given responsibility for breaking bad news:

Which must be an awful job for them ... it must be hard, a lot of the times they can't say anything to them can they?

Interviewer: No.

Which I think is a good thing that we can, we're not leaving them.

This openness to feelings came at a cost which was described openly by many of the nurses as examples of LR.

> I think you have to be quite a stable personality to cope with the ups and downs. I think people can look [at] the fertility nurse and think 'nice clinic job, and like outpatients' which it is certainly not ...

> Interviewer: No.

> The highs and lows are probably more than anything I've ever worked in before.

> Trying not to be too down about it but being honest. It's really the best thing to do but be positive about it as well if you can. Knowing you can't do anything and ... they've got to accept responsibility for themselves, they're grown-ups at the end of the day. It's a big thing for them in their life and passing it back to them as well because it's hard for you then to accept all this responsibility for everybody.

Far less experienced nurses, e.g. the NQNs in study 2, were also able to describe productive recontextualisation which arose from learner recontextualisation.

In the following extended data extract (Box 7.7), the NQN describes productive recontextualisation as she reflects on the knowledge she had of being a *new* NQN working with HCAs who might have been in post for 10 years or more and how this affected her confidence as an NQN. The LR comes from her learning from her own experience, finding somehow the energy and motivation to change her behaviour and change the knowledge she uses about team working and working with experienced HCAs in different situations. She begins a new activity in a new situation, producing new knowledge and consequently, confidence in her abilities. She firstly describes recognising *feeling intimidated* and how this motivated or prompted her to change her behaviour. She then describes changing from '*begging*' HCAs to do tasks, being '*scared to ask someone to do something*' to being confident in her role as shift leader or coordinator and instilling a different and more team-based approach to working, '*learning how to handle different people*', '*I tried to show them well I'm actually working with you as a team*'.

> ## Box 7.7   Productive recontextualisation in newly qualified nurses
>
> At first it was really difficult because I was working with healthcare assistants who have been there for like ten years and like they know you're new and they will try to intimidate you I'm not going to lie, like you know, like at times you get to a point whereby you know your patient, you know what you're meant to do and then they start telling what to do if you know what I mean and sometimes you would end up like doing this yourself, but I think it's more of
>
> *(Continued)*

learning who you're working with and learning how to handle different people if you know what I mean and I've grown to learn, I've grown to learn that.

Do you think something could prepare you for that experience, because I think a lot of newly qualified nurses really, you know, they do struggle with this.

Sometimes I even used to just beg, like I'm begging someone, 'can you please help me do this', no it's like [they say] it's not their job you know. [I was] just begging because they've been there, you know they feel like you know you shouldn't be asking them to do things but I mean, and sometimes I'd even be scared to ask someone to do something.

Yeah, I'm not surprised. So how, how have you kind of learnt to deal with that aspect of it, have you changed your ways?

I have yeah, I think as you continue to learn, to work with people, you do learn them and also try to, I mean for me I tried to show them well I'm actually working with you as a team, I'm not your boss if you know, so I think if you try to show that I'm actually working with you, we are a team, then I think you get more from trying to 'can you do this', 'can you do this', if you show that you know, you're really helping me, we're helping each other then you know, I think you achieve more from delegating.

Later she describes in even more detail how challenging learning to be in charge was for her by talking about her panic and having to contain the panic and not let patients or HCAs know you're panicking:

Yeah, because it doesn't help anybody to, to get flustered.

Yeah, because if you panic and you show it and the patients are looking up to you to expect results, the healthcare assistants you know are calling on you, expecting you to help, if you show them that you're panicking they're going to panic, the patients are going to panic, the relatives are going to panic, you know, and it won't show a good picture. If you don't panic and ask for help, sometimes I go and call and you like, phone X and told her 'listen, this is going on and ...' yeah.

Of course, and then in the middle of that you had your, your assessment then.

Exactly [laughs].

It was just, in the midst of all of that.

Exactly [laughs], hmmm.

Conclusions

We have illustrated LR in a range of nursing workplaces in this chapter from studies 1–5. LR concerns the personal aspects of learning, skills acquisition based on a range of workplace or clinical experiences the student is exposed to, their prior learning as learners in their professional and personal lives, their life experiences and their orientation to lifelong learning and their engagement with lifelong learning as a praxis. What are the implications for nursing from these illustrations of LR? Is LR something we consider in nursing currently in curriculum design, in workplace learning models?

Our illustrations have shown numerous examples of LR in a range of workplace (clinical) settings from among student nurses and NQNs to experienced and senior nurses. While it may be true that the NHS struggles with sustaining at the institutional level itself as a learning organisation (Melia, 2006), it is clear that individuals develop a lifelong learning orientation to work and their professional lives. Our data also show that while LR occurs in the challenging context of health workplaces, it depends on a number of important supporting factors. These include:

- 'Time and predictability' where the lack of continuity in learning afforded by the nature of the work means competency and fluency in skills are hard earned. It may not be unusual that a student nurse or nurse might encounter one episode of a particular condition or procedure during three years of education but be expected to 'hit the ground running' on qualifying.
- Gradual release where the busy nature of the workplace and the focus on patient safety means that learning through mistakes is not allowed and the fast pace of the work relies on competency not learning at any particular crisis point.
- Enacted conversations where the hierarchical relationships between students and mentors militate against these learning opportunities and where the onus on qualified, experienced staff is to present themselves as competent and capable rather than engaged in learning.

LR is contingent upon the resilience of the individual and the context in which they work. In addition, we suggest that we have yet to confront the potential for LR in nursing education. We are just beginning to explore how students' personal histories and life experiences, including their cultural habitus and exposure to lifelong learning, shape their access to learning and thus predict their success in professional learning. Students' ethnicity and access to learning resources is particularly important here.

Another feature of our data is the importance of positive experiences of learning for LR to develop. Negative experiences in workplaces connected to hierarchical social structures and processes continue to mean that students learn to 'shut up and put up'. This may be important if the learning milieu is not inclusive, or doesn't feel inclusive to students. Barriers including structured, direct, indirect, conscious and unconscious racism are implicated here as Helen's work on barriers to overseas migrant nurses' learning shows (see Box 7.1).

It is striking that the examples of LR we include here show how important it is to consider the spatial associations between sites of learning. It is well established that the theory–practice split in nursing sets up a tension between sites of learning; this is what people in nursing education refer to as the hidden curriculum or the theory–practice gap. Nursing students are particularly affected by this aspect of LR. Their sites of learning are shared between the university, a constantly changing workplace (clinical placement) and their life circumstances. We prefer to call this the theory–practice split as we believe it is actively recreated both individually and at the institutional level. As a result, this tension between sites of learning makes LR difficult for nursing students. These sites of learning have become more complex as students' backgrounds on entering their pre-registration programmes are more diverse; they bring with them more diverse life experiences, greater responsibilities outside their studies. The pandemic in 2020 has brought into focus how isolating learning can be for all students. As a result, the theory–practice split may be even more complex than formerly imagined.

Finally, our data show how agency is an important feature of LR in nursing students and qualified, experienced nurses alike. Agency is not well studied in nursing education; despite the rhetoric of self-directed learning, we still police our students in their learning hours and their attendance. We police their attitudes, their behaviour while in university and workplace, their time-keeping and the way they dress – really, what we're asking in an old-fashioned sense, is are they developing into a good (female) professional? This surveillance makes agency rather a problematic concept and perhaps explains why one or two of our research study participants struggled with finding their voice and becoming effective learners.

In Chapter 8 we develop these points and those made in the conclusion in Chapters 5 and 6 to argue for pre-registration nursing education and continuing professional development models which are founded on lifelong learning, recognise the need for spaces for learning (including liminal spaces and threshold concepts) in health workplaces and the tension between sites of learning as a split which is actively reconstructed. These models should recognise through both LR and WR the need to develop nurses as knowledgeable practitioners in a process that is incomplete and never finished as all knowledge is provisional and identity development a lifelong process.

8

A new relationship between nursing knowledge, theory and practice

Chapter objectives

- Consider the findings presented in this book
- Critique grand theories in nursing
- Discuss the relationship between nursing theory and practice – revisiting the theory–practice split
- Set out the need for nurses to develop a professional identity which is inclusive of lifelong learning

Introduction

In this chapter we suggest a new relationship between nursing knowledge, theory and practice. As we emphasise throughout this book, nurses theorise in practice in creative, agentic ways. We therefore build on the findings we've presented in Chapters 5–7, where we argue that nurses don't *apply* theory in or to practice but recontextualise knowledge and develop local theories for practice.

We discuss how our work builds on McKenna's discussion of practice theory and the development of person-centred nursing theory (Manley et al., 2011, 2014; McCormack and McCance, 2010; McCormack et al., 2008). These writers argue for an emancipatory relationship between knowledge, theory and practice for nurses. In so doing, they address the gap between grand theory and current nursing practice (Manley et al., 2014). The practice development movement which informed person-centred theory was hugely important in articulating a professional vision of nursing as well as a theoretical framework. These authors, like us, see nurses actively constructing local knowledge. We build on this work by reframing the theory–practice gap to a theory–practice split which, we argue, is continuously reproduced in everyday practice both in academic and clinical nursing. We draw on theories of learning to show that nurses, like other healthcare professionals, are lifelong, agentic learners who rework knowledge in and through local practice. Recontextualisation theory allows us to illustrate how theorising takes place as learning. Our findings show how nurses adapt to changes in healthcare practices as they evolve, redefining their roles and building local knowledge to inform practice.

The findings in this book

Our argument in this book has been that nurses theorise in practice as active learners who continuously rework or recontextualise knowledge to produce new knowledge which meets local conditions. A key feature of their theorising is their ability to rework their existing knowledge and produce new knowledge for their (local) practice. They also show an impressive ability to manage ambiguity, complexity and conflict. These data show how all grades of nurses think about the reasons why they care in particular ways; they articulate to each other the rationale for the care they deliver; they think through ethical practice and their own learning preferences.

A distinctive feature of the study 3 data is that the staff we interviewed were not only nurses; they included occupational therapists and social workers working in new interdisciplinary teams. We have included data extracts from some of these HCPs as their struggle with new ways of working, their learning and theorising, mirrors the nurses' struggle and was synchronous with it too as we collected data. Additionally, this synchronous theorising about the nature of their work questions the claim that each profession had a distinct body of knowledge.

Our findings show that learning to adapt to the context in which nurses and HCPs work depends on a number of factors: their colleagues, their mentors, their own sense of agency and resilience as well as the busyness of the service. Their resilience is shown in their ability to learn and theorise even if they feel under pressure or simply too busy; even when they're dropped in at the deep end and forced to sink or swim. Nurses and HCPs show purpose and leadership and manage to sustain learning despite students feeling their learning needs are not always acknowledged and staff finding supervision of students challenging. Our findings show poor learning environments where evidence of knowing (know-how), tacit and procedural knowledge is present in clinical practice but know-that knowledge can appear to be absent. However, even in these circumstances, students learn and theorise through negative incidents as well as positive in response to challenging contexts of care; although not all negative incidents result in learning. It is unclear whether these habits of learning can be attributed to the ways in which the organisation explicitly fosters learning. And whether the foundations, dispositions and identities in early career nurses for learning and the extent to which learning is sustained in the unique ecologies of learning and practice (Barnett and Jackson, 2020) of the NHS continue. We argue learning may be sustained, based on the findings we've presented in this book which show that nurses and HCPs theorise as lifelong learners across a wide range of careers and specialities. Theorising in practice is part of a lifelong process of becoming knowledgeable practitioners. Knowledgeable practice is practice that entails the exercise of attuned and responsive judgement, when individuals and teams are confronted with complex tasks and unpredictable situations. Knowledgeable practitioners are constantly developing as multiple forms of knowledge are put to work and judgement is exercised in challenging contexts that are characterised by uncertainties and interdependencies The development of the knowledgeable practitioner is usually approached either from the perspective of the learning individual or the perspective of the social organisation of learning (Evans, 2017, 2020). We argue such development is better understood in social ecological terms that keep both in view through a focus on and understanding of the interplay of macro-, micro- and meso-level influences and how these change over time, and the dynamics of nurses' long-term learning and development.

A note of caution is necessary here in 2021 as we face the aftermath of the Covid-19 pandemic (and perhaps its continuation beyond 2021). The pandemic has increased levels of anxiety among health and social care staff (Ayling et al., 2020) as well as increasing their exposure to psychological stress and distress (Greenberg and Rafferty, 2021). This exposure will have provided multiple opportunities for staff to experience trauma which may lead to post-traumatic stress disorders. In the context of increased exposure to trauma and higher than normal levels of anxiety and stress, health and social care staff may have less energy and capacity for learning and sustaining learning ecologies.

The effects of the interplay between personal agency and the contexts in which nurses and HCPs work in the NHS on learning should not be underestimated (Jackson and Barnett, 2020). The NHS's ability to deliver an effective health service is above all decided politically, shaped by the government of the day. Policy changes result in reorganisations which affect staff's interpersonal working relationships, such as the forming of new teams and where they physically work; their conditions of work, such as new contracts; new targets which prescribe actions and activities and constrain flexibility for individual thinking and autonomy. This was evident in studies 1, 2, 3 and 5 particularly; it was less evident in study 4. This study collected data in a private unit which seemed to be an oasis of calm where change could be implemented thoughtfully and carefully. The environment in which these nurses worked was constructed and supported through integrated nursing and medical leadership. It allowed them to build knowledge and expand their practice individually knowing they were supported in doing so. Hence, they were able to explain their expanded roles and the everyday enablers and constraints in terms of the relationships between themselves and their professional colleagues.

Contexts are not 'backdrops' for agency but constitutive of agency. The organisation, work team or individual can be taken as the point of departure. Furthermore, each individual's personal history can be considered a platform for their coming to know and making sense of what is encountered in workplaces and in their wider professional lives. This sense-making process both shapes and reflects the person's intentionality and agency in the ways in which they engage with work roles, as shown recently by Vähäsantanen et al. (2017). What learners make of these recontextualisation processes also varies according to their personal characteristics and the scope for action that they have, individually and collectively, in any particular environment. Together with their prior learning and tacit knowledge, opportunities and affordances for learning may be unequally distributed (see Evans et al., 2004, 2006). Learner recontextualisation takes place through the strategies learners themselves use to bring together and put to work different forms of knowledge they have gained through the programme, through working with learning partners in college and workplaces and by observing, enquiring and working with more experienced people in the workplace. Mentors and other members of the team assist learning by providing opportunities to work at the next level and thereby providing learners with a more holistic grasp of the connections between aspects of practice (Hökkä et al., 2017); learners feel stretched through such activities and challenges. However, negative experiences in workplaces connected to hierarchical social structures and processes continue to mean that sometimes students learn to 'shut up and put up'.

It is striking that the examples of LR we include in this book show how important it is to consider the spatial associations between sites of learning in nurse education. Nursing students' sites of learning are shared between the university, a constantly changing workplace and their life circumstances. As a result, a tension is created between sites of learning which makes LR difficult for nursing students. These sites of learning have become more complex as students' backgrounds on entering their pre-registration programmes are more diverse; they bring with them more diverse life experiences, greater responsibilities outside their studies. The pandemic in 2020/2021 has brought into focus how isolating learning can be for all students. As a result, the theory–practice split may be even more complex than previously imagined.

The findings presented in this book illustrate that nurses continue to learn and theorise across their careers and in a range of roles, from student nurses to senior nurses in commissioning roles. We have presented data which show students' and NQNs' learning as they negotiate the theory–practice split as early career professionals and begin to recognise their learning in practice. In study 3, which is located in the community during a period of organisational restructuring, we show how teams of experienced mental health nurses, social workers and occupational therapists discuss the place of theory in multidisciplinary teams. We describe the roles of nurses working with long-term mental health conditions in the community and their negotiation of their changing roles in multidisciplinary teams as they struggled to articulate their purpose. The HCPs in this study were uncertain of their particular profession's future in the recent workforce configurations. What emerges is a sense of shared vision *within* multidisciplinary team members with associated professionally shaped philosophical perspectives, alongside a unique professional, disciplinary knowledge which develops from and informs practice. As Donaldson and Crowley argue (1978), a discipline offers a unique perspective on phenomena relevant to nursing. McKenna (1997) argues that to be a discipline we don't have to have a unique body of knowledge, but we do need to use any knowledge we draw on in a unique way. McKenna uses *apply*; we would prefer *rework* as we have argued in the preceding chapters, as *apply* infers that knowledge is simply transferred whereas we believe (and show) that new knowledge is constructed through recontextualisation. The fixation with whether nursing has a distinct disciplinary knowledge has hampered theory development despite hints in early writers' work that practising nurses in practice might contribute to such work. For example, McKenna (1997: 96) cites Dickoff and James's (1968) statement about their theory of theories to say that this 'led nurses to realise that they, as practitioners, could make a contribution to the formulation and use of theory'. However it wasn't practitioners who introduced grand theories to the UK, as Helen's experience in the 1980s makes clear – her introduction to grand nursing theories and models was through academics as was fairly typical across the UK (see Chapter 1). This was because grand theories were based on an empiricist and deductive philosophy as McKenna (1997: 45) argues. In other words, they were understood to be derived from research by academics to be applied in practice rather than be derived from practice to formulate theory. He cites Kikuchi and Simmons (1992: 2), who argued that as nursing theorists were empiricist and tried to be scientific, the 'upshot was that the knowledge being developed was fragmented and ununified' for nurses. It wasn't until the emergence of nursing practice development units in the 1980s that practising nurses were encouraged to develop local theories of practice but this was located in a few units only in the UK (Gerrish, 2001). Our findings show that nurses and their health professional colleagues more widely are able to integrate unified, disciplinary and multi-professional knowledge in their practice.

Our findings also show how traditional framing of nursing theory, grounded in nurses' philosophical beliefs around the person, the concept of health, the societal environment in which the person or patient lives and the definition of nursing as an act of caring, has been adapted by individual nurses who theorise to make sense of new working contexts. In many new roles, nursing activities vary from influencing care delivery, to organising care or to researching into care. These reframings shape our fundamental philosophical beliefs about the nature of nursing. The findings from study 5 show a reframing of the domains of nursing in the context of workforce changes where commissioning nurses do not directly deliver care but commission care. Commissioning nurses' focus is population health not individual health. The findings show that this reframing produces tension both for individuals and for how they are perceived by their practice colleagues. As Drevdahl and Canales (2020) argue, nurses and the public perceive a 'real' nurse to be an acute care nurse, not a nurse who plans, manages, evaluates or commissions care. This can be problematic for a nurse's identity and self-esteem. The findings in study 3 also show a reframing as nurses, social workers and occupational health therapists reframe their thinking around disciplinary knowledge. This reframing suggests that professionals can hold a tension between unique disciplinary knowledge, that of the health visitor or OT as well as interdisciplinary knowledge which enables them to work in teams in primary care.

Our findings show numerous examples of LR in a range of workplaces among student nurses, newly qualified nurses to experienced and senior nurses. While it may be true that the NHS struggles with sustaining learning at the institutional level (Melia, 2006), it is clear that individuals develop a lifelong learning orientation to work and their professional lives. Our data also show that while LR occurs in the challenging context of health workplaces, it depends on a number of important supporting factors. These include:

- 'Time and predictability' where the lack of continuity in learning afforded by the nature of the work means competency and fluency in skills are hard earned. It may not be unusual that a student nurse or nurse might encounter one episode of a particular condition or procedure during three years of education but still be expected to 'hit the ground running' on qualifying in a range of clinical situations.
- Gradual release where the busy nature of the workplace and the focus on patient safety means that learning through mistakes is not allowed and the fast pace of the work relies on competency at any particular crisis point, not learning.
- Enacted conversations where the hierarchical relationships between students and mentors militate against these learning opportunities and where the onus on qualified, experienced staff is to present themselves as competent and capable rather than engaged in learning.

In all five studies, nursing theory in practice is local and emerges to fit the context; we argue that nursing shares knowledge and draws on a range of disciplinary *knowledges* to articulate its purpose and practice knowledge. There seems no evidence of a grand nursing theory or models. On the contrary, our findings suggest that local practice theory is produced through professionals theorising in and on practice.

A critique of nursing theories

Simply put, theories of nursing are frameworks which may be used to direct nursing plans and be used to plan patient care. As new situations occur, such frameworks provide a means to investigate new circumstances, make decisions and manage new nursing care plans. However they have too often been used to structure communication with other nurses and the multidisciplinary team; perhaps even with relatives? They've been used to assist the development of nursing values and goals and to define the different particular contribution of nursing with the care of clients. Erroneously in our opinion.

In view of our findings, following Murphy and Smith (2013: Vol. 2), we argue that grand nursing theories and models should be seen as a phase of nursing theory development which helped the profession articulate its voice. They were developed in a healthcare system very different from our own in the UK; that is, a private health insurance system with limited publicly funded provision. They don't really help us understand practice in a publicly funded system of healthcare (albeit increasingly, a mixture of public and private funding). The positioning of nurse theorists in the USA is also framed by the market with the self-promotion of each academic's particular brand of nursing theory. As McKenna states, there is an 'ideology of grand theorists Parseans, Rogerians, Watsonians, worshipping their own particular gospel' (1997: 128).

In addition, each theorist takes a particular perspective, i.e. interaction, needs, caring, and imposes this view of the world on both nurse and patient. This constrains how patients are viewed and nursed which is not reflective of the complex world of nursing in the UK, as Manley et al. (2014) have argued. Imposing a particular grand theory of nursing on nursing irrespective of context doesn't recognise nurses' agency for learning and theorising (Dewing, 2008; Jackson and Thurgate, 2011; Manley et al., 2009). While grand theories are patient focused and have the patient as a central domain, they're not person-centred; that is, they don't put the 'person in the patient' (Goodrich and Cornwall, 2008). Person-centred care is more than applying or adapting a nursing theory. In person-centred practice:

> Nurses and nursing staff provide and promote care that puts people at the centre, involves patients, service users, their families and their carers in decisions, and helps them make informed choices about their treatment and care. (Manley et al., 2011: 35)

Mid-range theories address some of the limits (in our view) of grand theories, the latter rarely being grounded in research. Mid-range theories are a set of related ideas that are focused on a limited dimension of the reality of nursing. They are therefore grounded in observations of everyday nursing practice which reflect the reality of practice. They are developed into theory through theory development processes like concept development, propositions, literature reviews, and quantitative and qualitative evaluations of the theory in practice. However while they originate in practice, they are shaped by the same empiricist tradition as grand theories as they follow similar processes of theory development. There are many mid-range theories in nursing, including a mid-range theory of comfort (Kolcaba, 2003), advocacy (Bu and Jezewski, 2007) and nursing presence (McMahon and Kimberley, 2011). Again, mid-range theories have been applied to practice rather than developing creatively from practice. This is because both grand theory and mid-range theories ignore that nurses theorise in practice to develop local theories of practice. By contrast, mid-range theories in the social sciences have tended more to reflexivity. For example, in reflexive sociology (after Bourdieu) a range of intellectual tools and empirical encounters are used with flexibility of theoretical and conceptual approach, to develop theory through critical enquiry.

As we have seen in the data we've presented in this book, nurses theorise irrespective of the academic discourse taking place in universities. But they may be shaped or influenced by knowledge they've been introduced to at university in some way. In study 2, NQNs' recontextualisation explicitly involved making sense of university teaching in new contexts. We conclude, following McKenna (1997) and Manley et al. (2014), that we should focus our attention on practice theory and theorising in practice in order to describe local theories in further detail. These descriptions would enable us to understand how, or if, local theories can be tested as mid-range theories.

Grand and mid-range theories don't adequately capture theorising in practice and local theories because they are predicated on a particular understanding of theory. Theory in this tradition is highly structured and purposeful. It identifies phenomena and the relationships between those phenomena in order that their interactions can be identified, classified, explained, controlled for prediction. Nursing models are the highest level of abstract thinking in theory development where relationships between phenomena in nursing practice are conceptualised but not tested. Grand theories are also highly abstract, define phenomena and identify laws of behaviour associated with phenomena of interest, but do not always lend themselves to testing in practice. Mid-range theories in nursing are less abstract, but are still based on concepts and propositions which can be tested in different settings. Early nursing theories were developed largely from within the natural sciences paradigm, later psychology and ethics of care. This paradigm remains popular in the contemporary world, not just the academic (Jackson and Barnett, 2020). While their work was informed by observations of the nursing world which they built up to general theories of patient and nurse behaviours, the level of theory was highly abstract and in many cases, untested. So while grand and mid-range theories follow the empiricist tradition, only mid-range theories are routinely tested in practice. Grand theories are empiricist as they assume that particular phenomena behave in predictable ways or laws which can be seen as general laws. Of course, the assumption that laws are immutable has been criticised within the natural sciences and debated within nursing theory. The nursing diagnosis and the evidence-based theory movements in nursing in the 1990s are further examples of the empiricist tradition in nursing.

Smith's (1994) edited book is a good example of this empiricist worldview applied to nursing. Each chapter presents a different theory applied to practice. Some are grand theories – Roy's adaptation model applied to breastfeeding advice for mothers of infants in neonatal intensive care; Orem's self-care deficit model in mitral valve disease; Neuman's system model applied to a patient with multiple sclerosis. Others are mid-range theories: a grounded theory study of decision-making in psychiatric services; a theory of touch. They attest to grand and mid-range theorists' empiricist view of theory – namely that it can be tested and applied. While grand theories, models of nursing and mid-range theories share a focus on domains of nursing, they don't explain, as recontextualisation reworked in nursing practice does, how nurses theorise in practice.

The extent to which nursing theory is shown or understood to be predictable is interpreted differently by different theorists and not all theorists would go as far as to say that all theories can be applied to all nursing situations (Murphy and Smith, 2013: Vols 1–3). As Chinn and Kramer (1995: 220) argue, a more qualitative definition of theory is applicable to nursing: 'careful and rigorous structuring of ideas that project a tentative, purposeful and systematic view of phenomena'. McKenna (1997) has a good discussion of debates around this point. We're not so interested in defining theory here but in what the ramifications of such a narrow definition might mean for what we observe in practice, namely, nurses theorising in practice.

The implications of the assumption that theory can be transferred to practice are that the nurse who applies any theory does so unthinkingly as the integrity of the theory/model needs to be upheld – otherwise it undermines the premise on which such deductive theories are built. Following the logic of nursing models and grand theories, to adapt the model or theory would contradict the understanding of theory the model of grand theory was based on in the first place. This problematises our data unless we adopt a more qualitative and inductive approach to theory as suggested by Chinn and Kramer; one which allows inductive theory to emerge from practice. As Chinn and Kramer argue (2011: 2), 'nursing practice as something more inclusive and broader than empirics is, in our view, critical for a practice discipline'.

The lack of uptake among nurses of grand theories may be explained by the changes we described in Chapter 2 about the ongoing curriculum wars over doing (skills) versus thinking in nursing. The return to a more skills-based curriculum in the 2000s was heavily influenced by the drive for achieving clinical throughput and targets apparent through a return to task allocation (Smith et al., 2012). Indeed, this was the main thrust of the Francis Report into failures of care at the Mid Staffordshire Hospitals Trust (Francis, 2013). Significantly, these debates in support of *doing* made no use of educational theories which refute the dichotomy between thinking and doing as we set out in Chapter 1. But there's another important way in which this focus on skills is damaging. It obscures the lack of time for thinking in practice in increasingly busy workplaces in the NHS. The nursing process, which was the predominant form of care delivery during the 1970s and 1980s, was a system which enabled and encouraged nurses to think *and* do as it's based on nurses assessing, planning and evaluating care. The nursing process had been largely abandoned by the 2000s due to the pressure to achieve targets. Task allocation in its new form, i.e. meeting discharge and bed targets and delivering trained nursing tasks (e.g. giving drugs), had been reintroduced. This involves a return to 'team' or 'sides' nursing (by which the work was divided into two separate 'sides' of the ward to which the nurses were then separately allocated) and a move away from patient allocation.

In our view, the final difficulty with the empiricist worldview which underpins nursing models and grand theories is the way it has contributed to reproducing the theory–practice split (see Chapter 1). We have argued in this book that popular thinking in nursing tends to criticise the gap, rather than consider it a potentially productive relationship. This has resulted in a devaluing of nursing as professional project as a whole (Fealy, 1999; Laiho and Ruoholinna, 2013). Perceiving difference between theory and practice in nursing as a gap that must be closed constitutes a lack of understanding that students learn across contexts, including academic, clinical, self-directed, and a lack of support for students' learning holistically.

The relationship between theory and practice revisited

Laiho and Ruoholinna (2013) suggest that theory and practice are vague terms which are nevertheless formulated in terms of a theory–practice distinction (Nieminen, 2008). Underpinning this distinction is the belief that education and work are significantly different learning contexts (Smeby and Vågan, 2008a) and that each have their own valued knowledges which are somehow mutually exclusive.

Some would argue that there aren't knowledges in practice; i.e. that if we accept there are different knowledges, we accept there are different ways of looking at a patient problem which infers chaos and indecision (Kermode and Brown, 2011). For further reading here, see Rolfe (1999, 2001) and Kong (2004).

These beliefs are continually reproduced as the theory–practice split, as we argue throughout this book. The theory–practice split in professional education depends heavily on a belief that education and work are significantly different learning contexts (Smeby and Vågan, 2008a, 2008b). Laiho and Ruoholinna (2013) argue that the theory–practice split (which they call a gap) is an expression of the issues and problems that arise in connection with the expectations of the professional fields towards 'their' sciences. This is not made any easier in nursing because we draw on such a wide range of knowledge and learn in many different learning environments and contexts. Theory applicable for one context is unlikely to be appropriate for all other contexts in which nursing is practised.

The theory–practice split manifests itself in many different ways in nursing. It has been described as a *mismatch* between nursing as taught and nursing as practised (Gallagher, 2004). Allan et al. (2011) describe it as an interference in the partnership between universities and clinical context. It can also be manifested in the difficulties of integrating nurse education into higher education, especially in the traditional university (Smith and Allan, 2010; Spitzer and Perrenoud, 2006). Heggen (2008) argues that in some disciplines, including nursing, social work and primary school teaching, academic knowledge has a relatively low value or status. She suggests that this is because their practice is inherently social. They are professionals who act in the social field – meet other people with their intentions and opinions – and therefore it is difficult to apply theoretical knowledge to predict or explain exactly what is happening when they work. Theories which aim to predict are likely to fail in these disciplines and as a consequence be devalued by the professionals in practice in these disciplines.

To fully understand the relationship between theory and practice in nursing, it is necessary to examine how theory and practice is taught to nurses. The point at which and how a professional is introduced to theory or knowledge is important as it may set a relationship which informs later encounters with knowledge. In the UK, nursing students may be presented with a nursing theory textbook such as Aggleton and Chalmers' (2000) *Nursing Models and Nursing Practice* on the basis that nursing practice is underpinned, informed by and predicated upon nursing theory derived from nursing research. However grand theories are rarely research or evidence based. These are fundamental flaws which have been commented on over some considerable time by (amongst others) Wimpenny (2002), McCrae (2012) and Yancey (2015). And it is important here to note the impact for students in being introduced to two contradictory practices: evidence for nursing practice (taught as introduction to research or evidence for practice) and nursing theory (frequently introduced as grand nursing theories or models which generally have not been tested in practice). In Helen's experience, students struggle with the differences between grand theories (in their eyes, not evidenced-based but sometimes seeming to be based on values they identify with) and evidenced-based nursing.

If students are introduced to grand nursing theory, these orientate students to one dominant view of the patient, family, health, environment and the nurse's role which is largely normative (Allmark, 1995; Murphy and Smith, 2013). While there is nothing wrong in getting students to think philosophically about the nature of nursing, the nature of being a patient and health, seeing these experiences through one lens (the philosophical lens of a particular theorist) can seem remote from the practice nursing students witness in clinical placements. Grand nursing models can also seem over-prescriptive as they assume one theory applies in all nursing contexts.

One of the most common difficulties for nursing students is helping the student to integrate theory and practice both in practice and in college/university to form a coherent body of nursing knowledge. This is not infrequently an unsatisfactory process as students realise that what has been taught in university is not what is used or seen in practice. Jensen and Lahn (2005) point out that perhaps the student does not feel what has been taught in the university is relevant, or the student is actually told it is not relevant. Perhaps students cannot find evidence for caring activities, for washing or dressing patients, or indeed students are told it is sufficient to be kind and compassionate. Much of the nursing witnessed by nursing students in clinical placements is governed by custom and practice, or by organisational policy which means nurses learn to rely on protocols, which reduce critical thinking and thereby professionalism (Allan et al., 2008). This is fertile ground for an uncritical acceptance – a reification – of the theory–practice split. As a result of this split, the knowledge students create in practice goes unrecognised as it falls between the gap – of knowledge taught in the university and knowledge learned in practice and from their observations of other nurses.

Students can also be taught theory in nursing programmes through evidence-based practice and research skills (Billings and Kowalski, 2006). Learning research skills such as critiquing a research paper, searching the literature and understanding hierarchies of evidence are intended to help students understand the underpinning research evidence behind the nursing they deliver while on clinical placement. It is hoped that nursing students become critical practitioners in future who are able to sift evidence after searching the literature, and weigh possible courses of action from evidence. However, research has shown that research utilisation by practising nurses is low (Forsman et al., 2012; Meijers et al., 2006). The assumptions behind the concept of *hierarchies of evidence* is also strongly disputed generally (Kitson, 2002; Rolfe, 2005) and particularly so in nursing where many nursing tasks are orientated to developing relationships between patients, families and nurses and are not supported by or possibly conceptualised as evidence. Evidence for practice (theories based frequently in biosciences) is separate to knowledge nurses use in interpersonal relationships with patients, carers and families. The latter is grounded in the psychological and social sciences and seen as lower in traditional hierarchies of evidence. Unfortunately, many approaches to teaching theory or evidence-based practice in undergraduate nursing curricula do not articulate this clearly. Kitson (2002) takes this position further and argues that the evidence-based nursing movement is based on assumptions about the nature of nursing which are in tension with, if not in opposition to, person-centred caring and practice theories. A further difficulty with teaching theory as evidence is that there are different types of theory. Theories of hand washing, pressure area relief, nutrition, wound, and bone healing are middle-range theories and (hopefully) reflect what students observe in practice. Kitson (2002) among others argues that person-centred theories of nursing are not middle-range theory but practice theories which are, by their nature, local theories created by nurses in teams in local settings. These theories are excluded by a hierarchies of evidence approach to nursing knowledge and practice and suggest to students that theorising and knowledge production has no place in clinical nursing (Rolfe, 2005, 2006a).

Students may be taught to integrate theory and practice through the mastery of clinical skills in clinical skills laboratories (Morgan, 2006). These are designed to allow students to *literally* practise in safety with support from their clinical educators or teachers; this enables them to develop their psychomotor skills (Jeffries et al., 2002) and decision-making. The acquisition of skills is once again heavily promoted in the UK within the 2018 NMC Standards and in Standard 1.0 (Learning Culture) (2018b), 1.1–1.8 relate entirely to promoting safe learning but do not comment on learning from mistakes or challenging situations. Our findings show how important these learning situations may be for nurses (and any professional).

Teaching theory in clinical laboratories allows theory to be linked explicitly with practice skills in ways that cannot be guaranteed in practice where registered nurses acting as mentors have to balance patient workload and safety with the learning needs of their allocated students (Bugaj and Nikendei, 2016). Skills laboratories are used to teach essential skills such as communication, moving and handling as well as more complex skills such as handling equipment and catheterising patients; they are also used for 'skills and drills' to learn to react in clinical emergencies (Morgan, 2006; Ricketts et al., 2013). Learning in skills laboratories is predicated upon role-play, repeated psychomotor practice, observation and feedback (Haskvitz and Koop, 2004). Nevertheless, caution about how much the skills laboratory resembles real life is required (Morgan, 2006). As yet, robust, comparative evaluations of skills laboratories are few and far between.

Lastly, a word about balance between theory and practice in nurse preparation programmes. Over the years, nurse educators and practitioners have argued for either more theory or more practice (Evans, M., 2009; Morgan, 2006) as we show in Chapters 1 and 2. The current pre-registration professional preparation programmes in the UK balance learning across the university setting and clinical placements, where 50% is taught in university and 50% in practice. Universities and their practice organisations work in well-established partnerships to produce competent and caring registered nurses at all stages of the process, from interview to assessment. As Fealy (1999: 72) suggests, 'to practitioners and to educators the concern has tended to focus on efforts to achieve greater theory–practice integration, and more specifically, to promote practices which best express theoretical positions and propositions, principles and prescriptions'. This has had two effects. Firstly, where theory is not available, such as in caring practices, these activities have been reframed as nursing's moral enterprise encompassed in *Compassion in Practice Vision and Strategy* for nursing, midwifery and care staff (O'Driscoll et al., 2018a). Secondly, a concern with evidence has pushed nursing knowledge, along with grand theories of nursing to the margins and allowed person-centred nursing to be increasingly threatened.

Developing a nursing identity for future learning

Forming a work identity is an important step to determining the 'purpose and worth' of nursing (Willetts and Clarke, 2014: 165); to developing a sense of who one is and what one wishes to achieve as a nurse. Developing one's professional identity may be better thought of as an undertaking rather than an accomplishment. It requires a flexibility in thinking and an ability to tolerate confusion before understanding (Savin-Baden, 2020: 46). This is especially true in nursing given the competing disciplinary discourses about nursing roles and responsibilities (Drevdahl and Canales, 2020). As Drevdahl and Canales citing McBride (1996) state: 'Nursing is so equated in the public mind with doing procedures and giving medications that nurses who manage complex systems and conduct research are viewed by many as not being "real" nurses' (2020: 34). Note McBride's emphasis on the public's perception of nursing as *doing* rather than thinking or managing. Our findings show that NQNs, students, fertility nurses and primary care also struggled with being outside the mainstream nursing identity. For the GBNs in study 5, their new role appeared to be particularly uncomfortable; they tried very hard to reassert their nursing *credentials* to justify their role in the face of perceived judgements.

The formation of identity is made more difficult for nurses because of the struggle to identify exactly what nurses do; as the nurses and HCPs in our studies found. Nurses' work is *unseen and unrecognised* (ten Hoeve et al., 2013; Willetts and Clarke, 2014), invisible (Allan, 2001). This makes the formation of a professional identity an arduous process made worse because historically nursing has struggled to be seen as a profession by other professions (Davies, 1995). This struggle has been similar across other female dominated professions like teaching and social work.

Developing a professional or work identity entails individuals creating, fixing, or reworking the creations that give one a sense of unity and uniqueness (Sveningsson and Alvesson, 2003). An individual's work identity is not fixed after a course of study at the start of a career, but an iterative and lengthy process whereby an individual continuously forms and reforms their identity. It is the 'mutually constitutive process whereby people strive to shape a relatively coherent and distinctive notion of personal self-identity' within the context of their lives (Watson, 2008: 129) and for nurses and other HCPs, in the context of their workplaces which are subject to frequent change and reorganisation in the NHS. Identity formation is the result of complex interactions between agentic individuals and their workplaces, including their colleagues, managers and patients. These interactive social processes are key to identity formation, as who we take ourselves to be relies on what is reflected back to us (Watson, 2008). As Watson goes onto argue, we participate in and manage constructing identity through the 'stories' we tell ourselves and others about who we are (Watson, 2008). What is perhaps underestimated in identity formation is the effort individuals make to form their identity within their workplaces. This requires an agentic individual with an awareness of self in context – their place within the workplace and the dynamics of the workplace and the effects on them as developing professionals. Jackson and Barnett (2020: 1) argue that this interplay or interaction between self and context is best understood as a learning ecology where:

> Individuals are connected with a buzzing welter of phenomena, of media, of institutions, workplaces and social spaces, personal endeavours, and relationships, and fast-flowing swirls of information ... This configuration brings new experiences at least daily ... the act of learning is an ecological phenomenon that brings forth new meanings, and understandings of the world and of one's own being and identity in and with the world. The very act transforms us and the world around us. It is a learning ecology.

As our findings show us, it is crucial that professionals receive adequate support from the workplace as they develop professional identities. Vähäsantanen argues, citing Kira (2010), if professionals 'do not have the individual resources to engage in the continuous professional learning demanded, their well-being, satisfaction, organizational performance and commitment at work may be threatened' (Kira, 2010; Vähäsantanen, 2017: 3) and their identity development delayed. As we have seen, one of the features of learning in the NHS across settings and irrespective of career point, is the busyness of the work environment. The participants across studies 1, 2 and 3 argued that there isn't always time for the learning, either informal or formal, which Kira (2010) argue is key to identity formation. Professionals' comprehensive learning in both training and work settings needs to be fostered especially in the NHS where the learning for nurses is disintegrated (Allan et al., 2018).

The agentic processes involved in striving to become a knowledgeable practitioner have been explored in Chapters 5, 6 and 7. We have shown how agency, in putting multiple forms of knowledge to work, results in *adaptive* forms and *productive* forms of knowledge recontextualisation. The deepening of adaptive learning to productive learning accelerates theorising in practice where there are few pre-existing guidelines and where the development of attuned judgement in changing and unpredictable situations is crucial to effective practice. Newly qualified nurses come to embody knowledge cognitively and practically through agentic processes. Ontology and epistemology merge in understanding how nurses become knowledgeable practitioners, capable in their own eyes and recognised by the ward team.

As fully qualified practitioners move beyond the liminal newly qualified state, knowledge undergoes further recontextualisations as practice varies from workplace to workplace, from situation to situation, and over time as practitioners exercise and attune their professional judgement. Practitioner capabilities, changing relationships in reconstituted NHS teams and the wider challenges of rapidly changing and busier NHS services are interconnected in a wider social ecology in which the agency of the acting individual has many manifestations and possible outcomes.

The pandemic of 2020/2021 will require a shift in our thinking of how students and qualified professionals engage with learning in clinical practice, in the workplace. The demands of the pandemic have meant that the curriculum and models of workplace learning in the NHS have had to adapt quickly and responsively to ensure that the NHS has been able to redeploy staff and students. Students have volunteered to directly deliver care and have deferred their academic work in order to do so. These accelerated moves into frontline practice at a time of massive demands and uncertainty have been facilitated by the NMC as a regulatory body. At the same time, 'normal' routine work was for a time stopped altogether as the NHS coped with an influx of critically ill Covid-19 patients. Qualified nurses, who may have spent years in one clinical speciality, were moved into new areas with much reduced preparation time. These changes have forced the profession to accept previously unheard-of standards of training (for students and redeployed staff), supervision (of both students and redeployed staff) and ways of working (numbers of critically ill patients staff are responsible for on a shift; working in personal protection equipment for entire shifts). The profession has had to rethink the curriculum and how it is delivered; the sites of learning a student encounters have increased and the potential for competing values associated with those different sites of learning has also increased. Therefore, the arguments we have made in this book and discussed more fully in this chapter will be subject to refinement as we emerge from the pandemic. What is clear is that learning and professionals who understand how they learn, for whom learning is a core part of their professional identity, will be central to sustaining future workforce development.

Conclusion

Our argument in this book builds on McKenna's argument for practice theorising and person-centred care theory (Manley et al., 2011; McCormack and McCance, 2010; McCormack et al., 2008) by arguing that Evans et al.'s theory of recontextualisation offers a way to understand how nurses learn and thus how they theorise, and practice theory develops.

Successful WR depends on the capacity of the workplace to support learners to learn and develop identities and purpose. Given such opportunities and support, nurses and HCPs show how they reflect on their roles and activities, seek clarity about their purpose and develop leadership skills, namely, teamwork, being calm and organised, establishing a routine, working with others. Successful WR uses gradual release, time and predictability and enacted conversations to develop learners' ability to manage ambiguity, complexity and conflict. Nurses and HCPs in our studies show how they reflect on care and evaluate care they give as a routine part of their practice; they articulated to each other in handovers or in case conferences the rationale of what the nursing care is based on and use such opportunities for learning. And amidst such a busy workplace, they think through ethical practice.

In our discussion of LR we have emphasised agency as we see this as key to successful recontextualisation. LR is of course as important as WR and other components of recontextualisation, but nevertheless it is easily forgotten in an outcomes-based curriculum within a results-driven and marketised university sector. LR is contingent upon the resilience of the individual and the context in which they work. We suggest that we have yet to confront the potential for LR in nursing education. We are just beginning to explore how students' personal histories and life experiences, including their cultural habitus and exposure to lifelong learning, shape their access to learning and thus predict their success in professional learning. We are beginning to build into the curriculum expansive learning spaces where learners can think through their own learning preferences. Students' cultural and social capital including access to learning resources is particularly important here.

The findings from all five studies show that agency is a feature of learning for student and experienced nurses across a variety of clinical settings. However agency is not well understood or described in nurse education literature. We have suggested that this might be because old professional attitudes are still dominant in both clinical and university sites of learning. One or two of our study participants certainly struggled with finding their own voices, finding their own agency and becoming effective learners.

We have illustrated LR in a range of nursing workplaces in this book from studies 1–5. LR concerns the personal aspects of learning, skills acquisition based on a range of workplace or clinical experiences the student is exposed to, their prior learning as learners in their professional and personal lives, their life experiences and their orientation to lifelong learning and their engagement with lifelong learning as a praxis.

9

Concluding thoughts

Chapter objectives

- Discuss workplace expectations and disintegrated learning in nursing workplace learning models
- Think through the potential for liminality as a framework to inform identity formation in nurses across their careers
- Consider how ecologies of learning (Jackson and Barnett, 2020) might inform a new model for learning in nursing practice
- Reflect on how nursing education might embed learning from feelings

---

Introduction

In this book we have shown from research data that nurses are lifelong learners who theorise in practice. Our argument has been that the grand theories of nursing, models of nursing and mid-range theories of nursing don't explain how nurses theorise in practice. Thus our intention has been to rework recontextualisation in nursing practice. We have argued that recontextualisation theory provides a framework for understanding nurses' theorising in practice and illustrated this through our research findings. In this chapter we conclude our discussion of recontextualisation. We discuss the ways in which workplace expectations and disintegrated learning shape workplace learning in nursing. Then we suggest that understanding learning as a *liminal* activity might deepen our understanding of ways in which learners recontextualise knowledge and in particular, put multiple forms of knowledge to work as they form and reform their professional identities across their careers.

Liminal spaces are embedded in larger sets of relationships that influence the quality of the work environment and the practices of day-to-day work.

The organisation of work; professional, health sector workplace discourses; funding and industrial relations; and susceptibility to disruptive change, along with a worker's own sense of agency, all influence ecologies for practice and for learning. Keeping in view organisational, political, regulatory and cultural inter-dependencies – and how they change over time – potentially enables us to see social ecological possibilities for development.

Recontextualising knowledge is an agentic process that is subject to a combina-tion of proximal and distal processes. In the wider context of any large organisation, interdependencies of interests play out as senior managers exert influence over the culture of an organisation and its approach to supporting workplace learning. However, 'corporate' expectations are rarely transmitted intact into practice in large and complex organisations. Workforce development policies 'as espoused' at the top of the organisation often depart substantially from workforce development when enacted, and their intended effects may be far removed from those experienced, particularly at the lower end of the earnings distribution and in high pressure work-ing environments. These tensions themselves have to be understood as part of a wider dynamic, keeping in view the macro regulatory and policy environments and the interdependencies set up within and beyond the workplace. Workers and man-agers are engaged in multiple overlapping structures and 'communities of social practice' that can themselves be analysed in terms of interdependencies of processes and interests. How nurses recontextualise knowledge as they act through the chang-ing environments and relationships of work and work-related learning is discussed with reference to the contribution of an *ecologies of learning* approach (Jackson and Barnett, 2020). We argue that an ecologies of learning approach might make a difference to our understanding of workplace and learner recontextualisation and how learning in and through practice can best be supported.

In this concluding chapter, our intention is to start a conversation about learning in nursing from the premise that nurses theorise in practice. We argue that we need to reconceptualise the relationship between nursing knowledge, theory and practice. Throughout this chapter, we weave into our discussion what the implications of the illustrations we have given of WR and LR in this might be for the development of knowledgeable practice and practitioners in nursing. We end with some reflections on the possible longer-term implications of lived experiences in the 2020 global pan-demic for the evolving relationship between nursing knowledge, theory and practice.

Workplace expectations and disintegrated learning

Spouse (2001b) argues that clinical (practice/work) placements are integral for pro-fessional development in practice disciplines. A clinical placement assists the student in linking theory to practice. Jackson and Mannix (2001) contend that clinical place-ments provide nursing students with an opportunity to integrate theoretical knowledge whilst developing clinical skills. Note the words *linking theory to prac-tice* and *integrate theoretical knowledge whilst developing clinical skills*; these don't imply reworking existing knowledge to develop new local knowledge for practice.

In our view, the current models of learning in nursing practice lead to a disintegrated learning environment. We believe this is constructed by workplace expectations of students which act to constrain both student learning and lifelong learning in qualified nurses. A feature of the clinical placement for nurses and student nurses is that it is also a workplace in the UK. The NHS struggles to be a learning organisation because it needs to balance its work demands (based on patient need) with its teaching and learning requirements (Melia, 2006). Indeed, the 2018 NMC *Standards Framework for Nursing and Midwifery Education* make this very plain (2018b): safety of patients, staff and students is considered to be the most important standard. We have described in earlier chapters how the nursing work is also constrained by hospital or trust targets for patient occupancy and other targets throughout.

In this busy workplace, having a mentor who has realistic expectations of students in busy workplaces and knows the curriculum is important in creating good learning experiences for students. Mentors who have positive attitudes and motivations towards teaching and supporting student nurses' learning in clinical placements and perceive their mentoring role as part of their own personal and professional development as well as contributing to the development of the profession as a whole are a resource for students to succeed in clinical placements. However, mentoring may not be undertaken voluntarily and mentors may fail to connect clinical nursing with academic knowledge explicitly. This is likely to become more complex if, as Fealy (1999) argues, mentors *believe in* the theory–practice gap and thus implicitly behave as though theory and practice were disintegrated; in this way, mentors may reproduce a disintegrated learning environment for students as well as reproduce the theory–practice split.

It is worth adding here that even if the workplace is busy and mentors cannot spend time formally with students, students can learn from informal activities, simply from observing and interacting with experienced nurses in authentic activities (Taylor and Evans, 2009). One of the unacknowledged aspects of mentoring in nursing is the informal nature of learning potential in the mentor–learner relationship. Quinlan and Song (1998) describe this in the cognitive apprenticeship model where learners develop as members of a community of practice. Merriam and Caffarella (1999: 245) describe the outcomes of cognitive apprenticeship thus:

> First, learners internalize what they have learned to enable them to do the task or solve the problem on their own. Second, learners are able to generalize what they have learned to help them to apply their learning to identical contexts and to serve as a starting point for further learning.

Francisco (2020), working in teacher professional development, uses 'practice architecture' approaches that extend Vygotskian thinking (see Chapter 3 for our introduction to Vygotsky) to argue that when practices that support learning are interconnected to form a trellis, professional learning is better supported than when practices that support learning are isolated and do not interconnect with each other. Professional learning for newly qualified entrants in the workplace, Francisco argues, needs to be supported through site-based arrangements that will be most effective if they form a strong trellis of interrelated practices that support learning. This leads us to questions of the adequacy of mentoring in facilitating interrelated practices that support learning in nursing.

What should be the attributes of the mentor and their role in supporting learning, taking into account learners' zone of proximal development (ZPD) and the challenges of a lack of interconnection in practice architectures? The mentor works in the learner's ZPD as an experienced professional or journeyperson. Mentors can push the learner outside their ZPD to learn. The journeyperson's task is to provide:

> ... newcomers with a series of leading activities which, when carried out under their watchful eye, will take the newcomers just outside their current zone of development and cause them to re-think their current views and practices. (Lave and Wenger, 1991: 98)

Lave and Wenger refer to journeypersons as *old-timers* to represent experienced members in the workplace who are competent in their field: 'not the oldest members in the community of practice but 'those with the most expertise in the issue at hand' (Bockarie, 2002: 5). At times, when another journeyperson has more expertise in a particular field or task, the learner will observe them. This description of journeyperson points to a fundamental misapplication of the role of mentor in nursing, where the learner (student) is seen as a lower status subordinate and the mentor is solely responsible for learning activities in a supervisory rather than a learning support role. Mentors' training includes very little on learning but a lot on how to complete which forms required by the university at the end of the clinical placement. The role of the mentor has been formalised from what might be thought of in other disciplines as an informal relationship, through the incorporation of assessment into the mentor–learner relationship. In addition, students are not thought of as agentic learners who negotiate their learning as full members of a clinical team. The student in Chapter 5 who says: '*I decide what I want to do and who to be with*', was relatively rare as most students felt disempowered and passive in their learning (see Chapter 5). Largely as the result of curricula changes in the 1990s (see Chapter 2), they're seen as visitors to clinical placements rather than learners who are part of a community of practice: '*We don't have the time. Don't know where they learn why*' (Chapter 5). Finally, mentors are not journeypersons and many, having not been introduced to learning theories, are not focused on facilitating learning as such; many are pressurised by their employer to train as mentors very soon after registering as an NQN. Many simply do not have time to construct meaningful practice architectures with interconnected learning activities; nor does the busy NHS facilitate practice architectures.

Unsurprisingly, the mentor's contribution to student nurse learning may not always be beneficial and many students learn from negative experiences of being mentored (Pearcey and Elliott, 2004). Brammer (2006) suggests that the mentor may act as a 'gatekeeper' (in a positive or negative sense) to learning and the integration of theory and practice in the clinical learning environment, while students may perceive the assessment role to interfere with their relationship with mentors. The 2018 NMC Standards for Supervision and Assessment go some way to addressing this concern by introducing a supervisor role in place of the mentor and separating out the supervision and assessor roles in clinical placements.

So far, we've referred to mentoring as understood in pre-registration nursing programmes: a registrant who following successful completion of an NMC approved mentor preparation programme has achieved the knowledge, skills and competence required to meet the defined outcomes. However, where appropriate, we might also refer to a mentor and use the term preceptor, or guide, who would support learning for any nurse who was new to a clinical team and needed to achieve competence and knowledge in a new area or field of practice. The NQNs, fertility nurses and GBNs in studies 2, 4 and 5 are good examples of nurses whose new roles or changed working conditions required them to become learners in need of mentors in this sense. The fertility nurses in study 4 described a careful, mentored approach to learning in the unit as they developed expanded nursing practice roles. However, our findings from study 2 also showed that staff were busy and many expected the NQNs to be able to work as a fully functioning qualified nurse immediately after their initial period of supervised practice. There were neverless some exceptions of ward managers who tolerated NQNs' learning needs:

> ... we always say it will take you all of that time for you to sort of get to where you think, you know – you won't think twice about picking up the keys or you know, taking the ward or whatever, so that's the nice thing about the preceptorship.

Benson and Latter (1998) argue that the theory–practice relationship is shaped by politics in each clinical placement where students are allocated to learn. The political climate across all placements results from the hierarchy between staff who have knowledge and students who need to learn (Cahill, 1996). The students are dependent on staff to learn and to succeed. This hierarchy constructs two curricula, the formal and the hidden, which are opposing experiences that disintegrate learning and support learning for both students and their mentors (Field, 2004). Students and mentors may use clinical role-modelling, which allows a student to work with the mentor without any formal instruction but socialises the student into professional practice and local, political ways of behaving (Allan et al., 2011). The findings from study 1 showed how successful students become at negotiating learning opportunities. But it is essentially a disintegrated learning workplace, which is haphazard, unplanned and unsupervised. Working in this way shows the mentor that the student is willing to *'pull their weight'* and contribute to patient care without cost to the mentor on a busy shift. Clinical role-modelling also validates students' presence and experience in practice which the university fails to do (Cribb and Bignold, 1999; Spouse, 1998) further adding to the sense of disintegrated learning. Students learn that knowledge and experience gained in practice are professionally valued by their mentors while academic knowledge and theory are not.

Essentially, students are expected to provide labour and on registration are expected to be able to work immediately as fully competent nurses. Expectations of students and the lack of integration of theory and practice, the lack of preparation for practice and mentors' expectations of students form a learning context where students have to learn to negotiate their status as students in practice. Students have to learn in a disintegrated learning context where opposing values of learning exist. Allan et al. (2011) concluded that students learned despite the learning frameworks rather than because of them. Brammer (2006) also argues that students are proactive in constructing learning opportunities, as they cannot afford to rely on mentors as they are not the only keys to learning in clinical areas. Understanding the strategies that students use to draw out learning opportunities in clinical areas when mentors might be gatekeeping and not facilitating access is useful in identifying active learning and facilitating such strategies in preparing students for practice areas. Such strategies might form the basis of practice architectures and include interconnected activities of and for learning. Currently, students desire to fit in and be accepted by their mentors (Brammer, 2006) and mentors are more like patrons than learning guides. Brammer argues that negative experiences do not always reduce learning as some learning can come out of negative experiences; but when learning is negative and the student becomes demoralised, the focus on learning is lost as the feelings become paramount and interfere with learning (Brammer, 2006).

Liminality as a framework to inform identity formation in nurses across their careers

Liminality was used by van Gennep (1960 [1909]) to suggest a psychological or metaphysical subjective state of being at the threshold of two existential planes where a choice of direction is offered to an individual. Liminality describes key events during the life course when individuals (sometimes in peer groups) enter transitional phases from one social state to another (Allan et al., 2015b). Van Gennep described rites or rituals among small human groups which denoted these transitions as having three phases: separation/pre-liminal, transition/liminal and reincorporation/post-liminal. Liminality provides a conceptualisation of transition, transformation and fluency for learning (Savin-Baden, 2020). Liminal states are characterised by confusion and uncertainty; chaos in van Gennep's original description.

Identity work is key to professional development in nursing and identities are formed and reformed across a nursing career as nurses make sense of themselves in new contexts (Bosetti et al., 2012), workplaces, perhaps in a new role (Cook-Sather and Alter, 2011) or starting a course of study. Liminal states are not a once-in-a-lifetime event but a number of transition moments or journeys. Transitions have been described in many areas of nursing practice to conceptualise patients' transitions in illness (Lapum et al., 2012). In an early paper from study 2 (Allan et al., 2015a), we used liminality to rethink the messiness of NQNs' transition to competent practice. This transition was characterised by the NQN recognising herself as a competent NQN with her new identity formed. This was achieved through complex interactions between the individual NQN, her peers, her team, her manager, her preceptor and other significant colleagues in the organisation. Savin-Baden (2020: 46) describes a transition like this as a journey where a 'learner['s] engages[ment] with a liminal tunnel [through which it is] necessary to pass through liminal zones and move to a state of learning fluency'. Land et al. (2010) argue that liminal spaces occur when the learner is confronted with new forms of disciplinary knowledge or threshold concepts which are key to understanding disciplinary practice. Land et al. (2014) have proposed that threshold concepts are liminal states where the unsettling experience of crossing a threshold and reforming concepts leads to shifts in identity and potentially a sense of loss. However we argue that this cognitive framing alone gives insufficient regard to the social, embodied and interactional aspects of learning and the long-term work-life perspective of multiple transitions and development over time. While concepts are integral to practice, they are continuously recontextualised as practice varies from workplace to workplace and from situation to situation, as practitioners develop their capacities for professional judgement. Roles and relationships are continuously revised and re-enacted (Savin-Baden, 2020) as liminality is to be understood not only in cognitive terms, but also as ontological and multi-faceted.

Threshold concepts bind disciplinary knowledge together in a transformative way (Clouder, 2005) as the learner confronts existing knowledge; the learner is required to move forward, to exit the liminal state or tunnel, and must rework or recontextualise this knowledge. Of course, some learners may get stuck in the liminal state (Savin-Baden, 2020). The purpose of the liminal space is to facilitate a transformation of knowledge and identity. As van Gennep describes in other rituals of transition, as a result of learning within this liminal space, students emerge transformed in their knowledge. The professional/learner understands what is expected of her, how she learns best and with whom learning is optimum. A learner learns to become flexible in evaluating new knowledge, in interpretation of practice, in managing uncertainty, conflicting knowledges and different ways of knowing (as we see in our findings). Successful professional identity formation is contingent upon colleagues, mentors, leaders acknowledging and giving feedback on the newcomer's situation as a learner. Land et al. (2005) refer to threshold concepts as troublesome knowledge which accurately describes the feelings of uncertainty that transition through liminal tunnels evokes.

In Chapters 5, 6 and 7, we have explored learning generated through engagement with troublesome knowledge in work contexts. We have discussed how these practitioners rework knowledge within a transitional (liminal) space and what the process of becoming knowledgeable practitioners means in changing and uncertain contexts. The instances of WR and LR have highlighted interactions of people, experiences and spaces for learning, connected in a constantly changing dynamic. Moreover, knowledge changes as contexts change and new knowledge changes people, contexts and practices.

In our paper (Allan et al., 2015a) we suggested that NQNs learn to delegate to, and supervise, HCAs through recontextualising knowledge; and that this transitional process occurs within a liminal space. We argued that for NQNs, delegation and prioritisation are threshold concepts. On registering, NQNs begin to think and practise as qualified nurses as opposed to student nurses and they enter into liminal spaces to acquire mastery of their new roles and understand these threshold concepts in practice. On emerging from these liminal spaces, they understand the underlying 'tacit' games of enquiry or ways of thinking and practice inherent to the discipline (Land et al., 2005). In these liminal spaces they recontextualise knowledge to emerge regarding themselves, and being regarded by others, as competent NQNs. Our analysis of recontextualisation in liminal spaces in clinical practice is a way to understand spaces and processes which allow for rites, uncertainty and new knowledge. Conceptualising learning in this way allows an understanding of the shift from student to NQN and the associated interaction of people, space and experience.

Billay et al. (2015), drawing on Land et al. (2005) and Cousin (2006), argue that liminal states may also be understood as psychosocial spaces to explore the learning journeys of nurse practitioners.

We have shown in this book that identity work continues through nurses' careers across different clinical workplaces. These moments or transition points are liminal periods when lifelong learners progress through learning journeys. There appear to be different points at which nurses might meet threshold concepts which require them to transition to new identities:

- progressing through their pre-registration programmes (study 1)
- registering as newly qualified nurses (study 2)
- moving into new roles as a result of reconfiguration and organisation of services (studies 3, 5)
- expanding their practice within roles (study 4).

Jackson and Barnett (2020: 1) argue that the contemporary world 'obliges human beings to learn and keep learning across and throughout their lives in order to survive and flourish'. Successful learners are those who enjoy the challenge of threshold concepts; those who aren't successful are those who retreat into conservatism and defensively protect old ways of knowing and doing. Learning in liminal tunnels involves conflict, uncertainty and entry to a new identity (Savin-Baden, 2020). Successful learners are threshold learners (Savin-Baden, 2020) who enter liminal tunnels repeatedly over their lifetime. As we've seen, they recur as nurses progress through careers. Learners *can* learn that liminal spaces or tunnels are productive in developing a new knowledge, new ways of knowing and new identities. However, social conservatism is a striking feature of nursing in the UK (Currie et al., 2010; Davies, 2004; Walby et al., 2004). Nursing curricula are pretty traditional and stick with accepted educational dogma and so struggle to prepare nurses for liminal spaces; we generally fail to provide integrated educational spaces and opportunities where 'awareness, capability and capacity can be developed' (Savin-Baden, 2020: 57). While curricula innovations such as problem-based learning and expansive learning increase flexibility in the curriculum, these have not generally been adopted widely in nursing. Given the findings presented in this book, one can understand why. The theory–practice split, the busyness of the NHS as a workplace and the rigidity of thinking in the NHS about the role of learning vis-a-vis learning and the NMC's regulator role, make a flexible curriculum an aspiration. There remains a focus on instrumentalism and practice-based skills in the nursing curriculum which can be anti-intellectual. In many instances, nurse education both in the academy and the clinical placement does not facilitate transformational learning. Our next section on ecologies of learning may help us to understand why.

Ecologies of learning to inform a new model for learning in nursing practice

We referred to ecologies of learning in Chapter 5 and again in Chapter 8 when we discussed whether individual habits of learning can be ingrained and sustained in an organisation such as the NHS. As Evans (2020: 163) argues, 'the ways in which adults learn in the workplace and throughout working life are rooted in occupational contexts and personal biographies'. As we've argued in Chapter 2, factors such as the role of women in society, the search for an evidence base, technology, politics, war, the economy and the influence of medicine have shaped nursing's development as a profession for over a century. This has resulted in particularly rigid learning methods both in clinical placements and in sites of academic learning which haven't always facilitated learning. As we have seen, from our findings presented in this book, these rigid learning methods still struggle to support learning and students frequently learn in the absence of support. We have illustrated how, despite in some cases a negative learning culture and quite prominent barriers to learning, individual agentic nurses (and HCPs) become lifelong learners who theorise in practice. In further understanding professional learning, the challenge is to understand the interaction between the agency of the learning individuals and the structures, institutional processes, milieus and relationships that mediate their continuing learning and development as knowledgeable practitioners. An ecologies of learning approach allows us to do this (Barnett and Jackson, 2020).

Ecologies of learning allow us to illuminate and understand the dynamics of interactions between learners and their work colleagues, mentors, supervisors and managers within a broader social context than recontextualisation theory. These dynamics shape how WR and LR are enacted; how factors which determine recontextualisation play out. Factors such as: timing which allows practices to be predictable for learners, gradual release of activities and enacted conversations with mentors.

Ecologies of learning originate in the biological meaning of ecology: the relationships and interactions of organisms with their wider natural environment (Jackson and Barnett, 2020: 4). Within individual ecosystems, an organism constructs an ecology for living which sustains its fundamental needs, such as nutrition, sleep, reproduction and survival (protection). An ecosystem contains an infinite number of 'organism-created ecologies for living' (Jackson and Barnett, 2020: 5). This idea of ecology has been applied to human ecologies – 'the relationships and interactions between people and other organisms, resources and environments for the purpose of living' (Jackson and Barnett, 2020: 5, citing Lemke, 2000). All organisms adapt to changing environments to survive but human beings can creatively and constructively plan this adaptation; in other words, they learn to survive. Learning therefore is an inherent and significant aspect of human activity. Learning is an individual transformative process across different sites of learning, frequently contemporaneously. Jackson and Barnett (2020) ask how we may better understand as individuals and society how to manage our transformations through learning an ecological awareness of learning or understanding of ecologies of learning?

Ecologies of learning link people with their ways of thinking, being and doing in the environment (both locally and societally). An ecologies of learning approach argues that learning and environment are indivisible as much as learning is doing. In other words, individuals can't learn without doing and learning is itself practice. Each constituent component of the learning ecology has meaning and therefore value. Relationships and interactions in the ecology of learning continually shape and reshape value and meaning. Thus the learning environment is a site where new values and meaning and thus identity are formed. They allow us to think and act creatively through new relationships, materials and our environment. Ecologies of learning are present whether individuals or teams are aware of them or not; forming as people interact and learn implicitly from each other. They are also formed intentionally, agentically, and develop a structural element which exerts its powers on individuals. Finally ecologies of learning are embedded in social systems and therefore, any analysis of learning requires an analysis of the interaction between individual agency and social structures; between 'workplace practices and occupational environments that are potentially generative of learning without losing sight of the learning individual' (Evans, 2020: 163). In rapidly changing work environments, an examination of the dynamics of the whole system at play reveals the ways in which the human processes of working and learning are intertwined, as workers interact and develop practice, reworking multiple forms of knowledge to meet situations that demand responses. In the work environment, practice ecologies generate learning ecologies that can extend, produce, limit or undermine learning.

When professional learning is viewed as integral to the practice ecologies that give rise to it, attention has to be paid to the environment as a whole, the institutional meso-systems and the exo-system influences arising from educational partnerships and frameworks for formal learning/qualification. The quality of the work environment affects the scope for reworking knowledge in a transformative process learning through day-to-day activities. We have explored the scope for the mediation of different, sometimes competing, interests at the practical level. For example, supervisors under pressure of targets are often reluctant to find the time and space to allow NQNs to put new ideas that might have been sparked by enquiry, observation and reflection into practice.

In nursing it seems to us that there are fundamental problems with embedding and sustaining an ecology of learning. As we have shown, a disintegrated learning environment and conflicting workplace expectations lead to differing values between sites of learning for nurses. These include differences between the academy, the curriculum, the national regulator (the NMC), clinical placements and practice workplaces. These differences are based on differing values and meanings around learning and the nurse as a lifelong learner. They create disjunctions at the meso-level (O'Toole et al., 2020). These values, meanings and ensuing practices are produced and reproduced through relationships, interactions, objects and methods of learning. Perhaps the most important difference in value is evidenced in the theory–practice split which is premised on the belief that thinking and doing are different activities and learning is achieved through doing alone. If learning is doing and therefore separated from thinking, wholly embedded in practice itself, then learning in universities and other sites of learning (in voluntary work placements, through personal lives, online communities) may not be valued as learning and the learning ecology is therefore under threat because it cannot be sustained in a disintegrated environment. Nursing does not have the means (facilitative meso-systems) by which learning and experiences can be connected, integrated and (we argue) reworked across contexts and situations and over time. Rather, disjunctions at the level of meso-systems threaten the sustainability, and very existence, of a learning ecology.

Embedding learning from feelings in nurse education

In Chapter 8 we develop the points made in the conclusions in Chapters 5 and 6 to argue for pre-registration nursing education and continuing professional development models which are founded on lifelong learning, and recognise the need for spaces for learning (including liminal spaces and threshold concepts) in health workplaces and the tension between sites of learning as a split which is actively reconstructed. These models should acknowledge through both LR and WR the need to develop nurses as knowledgeable practitioners in a process that is incomplete and never finished as all knowledge is provisional and identity development a lifelong process.

Developing a lifelong learning approach requires staff being stretched through opportunities to work at the next level and thereby providing learners with a more holistic grasp of the connections between aspects of practice (Hökkä et al., 2017). Hökkä argues that as well as interest in professional agency, there is a need to understand how *emotions* are embedded in agentic practice. We have emphasised throughout the book the challenges to agency within the strongly hierarchical profession that is nursing. Our findings speak to nurses' resilience in the face of barriers to learning and an ecology of learning which is frequently dysfunctional. Hökkä et al. (2017) argue that emotions are intimately bound up with work and shape professional agency.

Drawing on Fabricius (1999) and Menzies-Lyth (1970), Allan (2011) has argued elsewhere that a student's emotional learning is a means to integrate theory with practice. Understanding emotional learning psychodynamically, or as Fabricius suggests, through learning to work with feelings in nursing practice, allows the nurse to recognise that feelings shape learning both consciously and unconsciously. Feelings are the fundamental basis of learning for students and nurses as they learn from interactions with patients, their families and colleagues. They shape interactions and therefore learning. Allan (2011) argued that using a psychodynamic approach in nurse education may address the theory–practice gap for student nurses by allowing them to reflect on the emotional issues arising in clinical placements. She showed how supervision can assist students to integrate theory and practice through guided reflection on feelings arising from their learning in placements in small group work with a skilled tutor who works psychodynamically. Learning to work with feelings means that, following Menzies-Lyth, the nurse is aware that as well as the clinical dimension of delivering care, there are also social and emotional processes at work in interactions with patients which affect how we feel (Fabricius, 1999). Sometimes we are aware of these feelings and can reflect *in* action – this means we are able to recognise the patient's feeling and our own responses, and act appropriately. Sometimes we can only reflect *on* action, i.e. after the event and learn from that reflection to work differently in similar situations in the future. This approach derives from Freud's theory of the individual's internal psychodynamic world (Fabricius, 1991, 1995). These feelings are frequently buried and although they shape action, are not processed or learnt from. Evans (2009) has described the theory–practice gap as a way (in psychodynamic terms) of keeping the messiness of learning under control when the nurse is with the patient. The student's learning challenges this control over feeling and messiness and leads to an unconscious split of theory from practice for students, nurses, educators and mentors.

Fealy (1999) proposes a typology to characterise the theory–practice relationship in nursing by drawing on Carr's (1986) assertion that one can describe these relationships as: the common-sense approach, the applied science approach, the practical approach and the critical approach. The recognition of different forms of theory and knowledge in nursing has been possible because of a rejection of the technical-rational approach to knowledge and its underlying assumption that theory informs practice rather than there being a symbiotic relationship. Since the 1990s, theorists have been concerned with understanding how nurses theorise in practice (Benner and Wrubel, 1989). In work over two decades, Benner et al. (2009) emphasise that students learn from experience where tacit knowing and intuition become critical skills to acquire expertise and that the acquisition of practical skills is a critical feature of and prerequisite for professional expertise. Many nurse theorists have argued for the use of critical reflection as a tool with which to create knowledge for practice (Rolfe, 2014). This is known as practice-driven theory – theory recoverable from good practice through reflection to guide practice. Central to practice-driven theory is *praxis* or the action of learning to change practice (Rolfe, 1993, 2006a). Through reflecting on practice while in practice, the nurse or team of nurses modify and develop practice. Critical reflection or reflexivity validates the professional judgements of practitioners. As a result, the theory–practice 'gap' disappears as theory is derived from and tested in practice. However, the knowledge and theory utilised in practice is local and situated. While local, situated knowledge is valid, this approach to knowledge and practice-driven theory may be too situational, too local (Fealy, 1999). In reality, there is place for both forms of knowledge and different levels of theory (Fealy, 1999): local situated knowledge which informs local practice and theorising; middle range theory which takes nursing practice beyond the local to inform nursing care such as wound care, pressure area care, mouth care. Even grand theory when appropriate in context.

Conclusion

It seems to us that current theories of nursing and theories of learning in nursing have led to a failure in nursing to:

- engage in debates about nurses as lifelong learners
- consider how nurses continually reform professional identity across their careers and how this contributes to knowledge development and theorising in practice
- critique the reification of the theory–practice gap and the lack of consideration paid to the reproduction of the theory–practice split in everyday nursing practice
- recognise that nurses theorise in practice and develop local knowledge for practice
- embed practice theory as the basis for nursing practice.

Most higher education degrees and diplomas that aim to prepare participants to work in a particular profession or occupational field now incorporate placements or periods of practice-based learning as part of the learning programme. Work-based learning components have proliferated with the expansion of new degrees and diplomas in areas such as agricultural technology and digital forensics. Sometimes essential periods of practice-based learning take place after the programme as the graduates take up positions that enable or require further workplace-based learning. For example, for legal careers, firm-based 'training contracts' offer periods of recognised practice-based training that are requirements for full entry to the profession; and, in commercial firms, structured internships in graduate training schemes often fulfil this function. In fields as diverse as aircraft engineering, finance, glass industry, media practice and public administration, the challenges of theory–practice gaps have become evident, as students, teachers, mentors and supervisors struggle to put the different forms of knowledge developed within and beyond the degree or diploma to work in new and changing contexts, as exemplar cases in Evans et al. (2009) have shown. Previous and current conceptualisations of the theory–practice gap in nursing fail to examine the nature of knowledge in a practice discipline. In so doing, they do not resolve the problematic relationship between knowledge, curriculum, learning and practice. In nurse education, it is typical for questions to focus on how learning can be 'transferred' from one setting to another, relating the assumed 'abstract' nature of theory to the assumed 'real' nature of practice. This is often seen as a single movement as encapsulated in the term 'from theory to practice' which is based on an assumption that thinking is not doing, that learning is not practice.

The most recent Nursing and Midwifery Council's Standards for registered nurses and for preparatory nursing programmes (NMC, 2018a) reinforce this split between practice and education, between thinking and doing. These Standards use words such as thinking critically and self-reflection to describe learning but not learning itself. There are references to demonstrating and applying knowledge and a list of different forms of knowledge including (as you would expect) physiology, psychology, policy, politics. But there is no description of what nursing knowledge might be or how it might be taught or learnt apart from through evidence-based knowledge for practice (NMC, 2018a, 2018b). In Standard 1.0 (Learning Culture) (2018b) there is no reference to even knowledge transfer at all. Reading the new Standards, it is as if not only is the theory–practice gap reinforced but that there is a structural divide between practice and theory.

If nurse lecturers and students could understand the potential for learning and theorising across sites of learning and in practice, nurses could articulate more meaningful local theories for practice and use local and mid-range theory to inform practice. Much of nursing's relationship with theory and the consequent theory–practice split is exemplified in Fawcett's definition of the relationship between theory and practice. While Fawcett describes the 'reciprocal relationship between conceptual models (theories) and practice' (1992: 64), she ultimately sees this as (more or less) a one-way street with theory informing practice as the dominant partner; practice may have some feedback to theory but essentially, theory should guide practice, in her view.

Nurse educators need to be quite clear that some nursing activities, such as dressing wounds, require theoretical knowledge. Other nursing activities are not underpinned by evidence and rely instead on knowledge; which could be empathic knowing, aesthetic knowing or knowledge about how to reflect and learn. As Allmark (1995) suggests, the type of knowledge associated with nursing practice should not be taught through theory, nor is it well represented in theoretical terms. The knowledge of the practitioner is not theory, but something else. We have argued that the relationship between theory and practice is a more symbiotic one where practice is based on *knowledge* rather than (nursing) theory, as Fawcett and others argue. Nurses build up local theories of practice based on knowledge reworked from other sites of learning.

We have explored, in Chapters 5, 6 and 7, how learning is generated through engagement with troublesome knowledge in work contexts. We have discussed how these practitioners rework knowledge within a transitional (liminal) space and what the process of becoming knowledgeable practitioners means in changing and uncertain contexts. The instances of WR and LR have highlighted interactions of people, experiences and spaces for learning, connected in a constantly changing dynamic. Moreover, we have shown how knowledge changes as contexts change and how new knowledge changes people, contexts and practices.

In the light of the pandemic in 2020/2021, we need to consider what happens when this dynamic is disturbed by massive, discontinuous change. As we suggested in Chapter 8, the pandemic has increased staff and students' anxiety and the potential for trauma as well as increased workload in the NHS. The focus has been on survival of the NHS rather than considering how we can learn from the challenges staff in the NHS have successfully negotiated. Learning from such massive changes might be challenging but the pandemic might also offer opportunities (Lambert, 2021). The pandemic has forced us to develop at speed online learning communities, blended learning strategies and methods and enhanced our online virtual contact with students. Student evaluations in the Adult and Child and Mental Health branches of nursing at Middlesex University are generally positive. Attendances at seminars, small groups and even lectures are better than at face-to-face sessions. This offers the potential for integrating sites of learning underpinned by agentic practices from students and fostered by lecturers who construct opportunities for such integration. Such practice architectures just might be possible. Our findings show that the NHS does facilitate learning in places and at times, that individual learners maintain a lifelong learning orientation throughout their careers and that teams can foster learning. Recontextualisation and an ecologies of learning approach might allow nurse educators to respond to the challenge of reintegrating learning in nurse education through innovative expanded learning in the curriculum in the wake of the pandemic. Potentially, pandemic responses in the NHS provide an exceptional (real-world) scenario to test digital technologies in nursing education and construct digital communities of practice.

Finally, we ask to what extent can our approach – focusing on the agentic processes of reworking knowledge while keeping in view organisational, political, regulatory and cultural interdependencies and how they change over time – enable us to see new possibilities for development? We have shown how, in nursing environments, an examination of the dynamics of the whole system at play reveals the ways in which the human processes of working and learning are intertwined, as workers interact and work together, constructing and developing social practices as many different forms of knowledge are put to work. We have also shown the tensions, contradictions and disintegrations that can occur when knowledge is not put to work at both levels of learner and workplace recontextualisation.

We have emphasised throughout that this book represents how ideas of recontextualisation are themselves being recontextualised in and for the nursing field. Other reworkings are in train in other fields, with researchers such as Rogers (2020), building on Evans et al.'s recontextualisation approaches in working with small groups of experienced adult professionals typically transitioning from specialist to enterprise roles. Rogers' approach, reworked for business contexts, has wider resonances in challenging assumptions about theory, practice, knowledge and learning. It also has unique features in highlighting temporality and developing interactive visual tools that aim to facilitate reflection on the relationship between learning and time in post-classroom ('real-world') settings.

The temporal dimension has been approached, in this book, through the notion of liminality. We have argued for enhanced social ecological understandings of liminal spaces for learning that bring into view the dynamics of uncertainty as well as professional development over time. We signal here the potentiality for further development of recontextualisation theory in exploring more fully the temporal aspect (i.e. the chrono-system in socio-ecological terms). Findings from our research studies suggest the temporal aspect of recontextualisation could be explored in relation to:

- new roles such as advanced practitioner roles being introduced across nursing and healthcare professions
- new mentor/supervisor arrangements for pre-registration programmes
- innovative curricula and teaching methods.

In the light of our findings, research could also be undertaken using co-production methodologies with staff and students into exploring how sites of learning can be integrated in nursing and other practice disciplines.

Finally, we suggest that social ecological perspectives facilitate the development of social imaginaries for nursing where nurse education may be imagined in new ways that fundamentally rethink learning and professional identity in the 21st century.

References

Abdal-Haqq, I. (1999) Constructivism in teacher education: considerations for those who would link practice to theory. *ERIC Digest*, June 1999. Retrieved from: Wisiwgy://58/http://orders.edrs.com/members/sp.cfm (accessed 20 November 2001).

Acheson, D. (1998) *Independent Inquiry into Inequalities in Health Report Chairman: Sir Donald Acheson*. London: Department of Health.

Aggleton, P. and Chalmers, H. (2000) *Nursing Models and Nursing Practice*. 2nd ed. Oxford: Macmillan.

Alderson, P. (2020) Powerful knowledge and the curriculum: Contradictions and dichotomies. *British Educational Research Journal*, 46: 26–43.

Allan, H. T. (2001) A 'good enough' nurse: supporting patients in a fertility unit. *Human Fertility*, 4: 18–23.

Allan, H. T. (2005) Gender and embodiment in nursing: the role of the female chaperone in the infertility clinic. *Nursing Inquiry*, 12(3): 175–183.

Allan, H. T. (2010) Mentoring overseas nurses: barriers to effective and non-discriminatory mentoring practices. *Nursing Ethics*, 17(5): 603–613.

Allan, H. T. (2011) Using psycho-dynamic small group work in nurse education: closing the theory-practice gap? *Nurse Education Today*, 31(5): 521–524.

Allan, H. T. (2016a) Becoming a patient. In H. T. Allan, D. Kelly, P. Smith and M. Traynor (eds), *Understanding Sociology in Nursing*. London: Sage. pp. 7–26.

Allan H. T. (2016b) Nursing the body. In H. T. Allan, D. Kelly, P. Smith and M. Traynor (eds), *Understanding Sociology in Nursing*. London: Sage. pp. 117–136.

Allan, H. T. and Barber, D. (2004) Nothing out of the ordinary: advanced fertility nursing practice. *Human Fertility*, 7(4): 277–284.

Allan, H. T. and Barber, D. (2005) Emotion boundary work in advanced fertility nursing roles. *Nursing Ethics*, 12(4): 391–400.

Allan, H. T. and Mounce, G. (2015) Managing infertility in primary care. *Practice Nursing*, 26(9): 440–443.

Allan, H. T. and Westwood, S. (2015) English language skills requirements for overseas trained nurses working in the care industry: barriers to UK registration or institutionalised discrimination? *International Journal of Nursing Studies*, 54(1–4).

Allan, H. T., Smith, P. and Lorentzon, M. (2007) Leadership for learning: a literature study of leadership for learning in clinical practice. *Journal of Nursing Management*, 16: 545–555.

Allan, H. T., Tschudin, V. and Horton, K. (2008) The devaluation of nursing: a position statement. *Nursing Ethics*, 15(4): 561–568.

Allan H T (2009) *Managing intimacy and emotions in advanced fertility care: the future of nursing and midwifery roles*. M&K Publishing.

Allan, H. T., Cowie, H. and Smith P. (2009a) Overseas nurses' experiences of discrimination: a case of racist bullying. *Journal of Nursing Management*, 17: 898–906.

Allan, H. T., De Lacey, S. and Payne, D. (2009b) The socio-cultural context of assisted reproductive technologies: the shaping of 'routine' practices. *Nursing Inquiry*, 16 241–250.

Allan, H. T., Smith, P. and O'Driscoll, M. (2011) Experiences of supernumerary status and the hidden curriculum in nursing: a new twist in the theory-practice gap? *Journal of Clinical Nursing*, 20: 847–855

Allan, H. T., Ross, F., Christian, S., Brearley, S., Byng, R., Smith, P., Mackintosh, M. M. (2014) People and teams matter in organisational change: professionals' and managers' experiences of changing governance and incentives in primary care. *Health Services Research Journal*, 49(1): 59–68.

Allan, H. T., Magnusson, C., Ball, E., Evans, K., Horton, K., Curtis, K. and Johnson, M. (2015a) People, liminal spaces and experience: understanding recontextualisation of knowledge for newly qualified nurses. *Nurse Education Today*, 35(2): e78–e83.

Allan, H. T., Bryan, K., Hunter, B., Knibb, W., Odelius, A. and Shawe J. (2015b) Gatekeeping access to the midwifery unit: managing complaints by bending the rules. *Health*, 19(6): 652–669.

Allan, H. T., Bryan, K., Hunter, B., Knibb, W., Odelius, A. and Shawe J. (2015c) Gatekeeping access to the midwifery unit: managing complaints by bending the rules, *Health* 19(6), pp. 652–669.

Allan, H. T., Evans, K., Magnusson, C., Ball, E., Horton, K., Curtis, K. and Johnson, M. (2016a) Uncertainty and the unexpected in clinical practice: invisible learning among newly qualified nurses. *Nursing Inquiry*, 23(4): 377–385.

Allan, H. T., Tapson, C., O'Driscoll, M., Savage, J., Lee, G. and Dixon, R. (2016b) A critical integrative literature review of governing body nurses on Clinical Commissioning Groups in the UK. *Nursing Inquiry*, 23(2): 178–187.

Allan, H. T., O'Driscoll, M., Savage, J., Lee, G. and Dixon, R. (2016c) A pilot study of governing body nurses' experiences on Clinical Commissioning Groups in the UK. *Nursing Standard Art & Science*, 30(42): 46–55.

Allan, H. T., Kelly, D., Smith P., and Traynor M., (2016d) (eds), *Understanding Sociology in Nursing*. London: Sage Publications.

Allan, H. T., Dixon, R., Lee, G., Savage, J. and Tapson, C. (2017) Nurses' experiences of Clinical Commissioning Groups: an observational study of two Clinical Commissioning Groups (CCGs) in England. *Journal Research in Nursing*, 22(3): 197–211.

Allan, H. T., Magnusson, C., Johnson, M., Evans, K., Ball, E., Horton, K., Curtis, K. and Westwood, S. (2018) Preceptorship and safe delegation: the key to improved standards in bedside care? *Journal of Clinical Nursing*, 27(1–2): 123–131.

Allmark, P. (1995) A classical view of the theory-practice gap in nursing. *Journal of Advanced Nursing*, 22: 18–23.

Avis, M. and Freshwater, D. (2006) Evidence for practice, epistemology and critical reflection. *Nursing Philosophy*, 7: 216–224.

Ayling, K., Jia, R., Chalder, T., Massey, A., Broadbent, E., Coupland, C. and Vedhara, K. (2020) Mental health of keyworkers in the UK during the COVID-19 pandemic: a cross-sectional analysis of a community cohort. MEDRxiv preprint submitted 13 November 2020. doi: https://doi.org/10.1101/2020.11.11.20229609

Barker, C., King, N., Snowden, M. and Ouse, K. (2016) Study time within pre-registration nurse education: a critical review of the literature. *Nurse Education Today*, 41: 17–23.

Barnett, M. (2006) Vocational knowledge and vocational pedagogy. In M. Young and J. Gamble (eds), *Knowledge, Curriculum and Qualifications for South African Further Education*. Cape Town: HSRC Press.

Barnett, R. and Jackson, N. (2020) Epilogue: practice seldom makes perfect but…. In R. Barnett and N. Jackson (eds), *Ecologies for Learning and Practice*. Abingdon: Routledge. pp. 223–229.

Barrow, J. and Sharma, S., (2019). Nursing Five Rights of Delegation. [online] Ncbi.nlm.nih. gov. Available at: https://www.ncbi.nlm.nih.gov/books/NBK519519/

Bassett, C. (2004) *Nursing Care from Theory to Practice*. London: Whurr Publishers.

Baxter, S. K. and Brumfitt, S. M. (2008) Professional differences in interprofessional working. *Journal Interprofessional Care*, 22(3): 239–251.

Benner, P. (1984) *From Novice to Expert: Excellence and Power in Clinical Nursing Practice*. Menlo Park, CA: Addison-Wesley.

Benner, P. and Tanner, C. (1987) Clinical judgement: how expert nurses use intuition. *American Journal of Nursing*, 87(1): 23–31.

Benner, P. and Wrubel, J. (1989) *The Primacy of Caring: Stress and Coping in Health and Illness*. Menlo Park, CA: Addison Wesley Longman.

Benner, P., Tanner, C. A. and Chesla, C. A. (2009) *Expertise in Nursing Practice: Caring, Clinical Judgment and Ethics*. New York: Springer.

Benson, A. and Latter, S. (1998) Implementing health promoting nursing: the integration of interpersonal skills and health promotion. *Journal of Advanced Nursing*, 27: 100–107.

Bentley, S. V., Peters, K., Haslam, S. A. and Greenaway, K. H. (2019) Construction at work: multiple identities scaffold professional identity development in academia. *Frontiers in Psychology*, 10: Article 628. https://doi.org/10.3389/fpsyg.2019.00628

Berg, E. E. B., Barry, J. J. J. and Chandler, J. J. P. (2008) New public management and social work in Sweden and England: challenges and opportunities for staff in predominantly female organisations. *International Journal of Sociology and Social Policy*, 28(3–4): 114–128.

Bernstein, B. B. (2000) *Pedagogy, Symbolic Control and Identity: Theory, Research Critique*. Revised ed. Lanham, MD: Rowman and Littlefield.

Billay, D., Myrick, F. and Yonge, O. (2015) Preceptorship and the nurse practitioner student: navigating the liminal space. *The Journal of Nursing Education*, 54(8): 430–437.

Billings, D. M. and Kowalski, K. (2006) Bridging the theory–practice gap with evidence-based practice. *Journal of Continuing Education in Nursing*, 37(6): 248–249.

Black, D. (1980) *Report of the Expert Committee into Health Inequality chaired by Sir Douglas Black*. London: DHSS.

Bliss, S., Baltzly, D., Bull, R., Dalton, L. and Jones, J. (2017) A role for virtue in unifying the 'knowledge' and 'caring' discourses in nursing theory. *Nursing Inquiry*, 24(4): e12191.

Bockarie, A. (2002) The potential of Vygotsky's contributions to our understanding of cognitive apprenticeship as a process of development in adult vocational and technical education. *Journal of Career and Technical Education*, 19(1): 47–66.

Bosetti, L., Kawalilak, C. and Patterson, P. (2012) Betwixt and between: academic women in transition. *Canadian Journal of Higher Education*, 38(2): 95–167.

Bound, H., Rushbrook, P., Waite, E. and Evans, K. (2014) *The Entrepreneurial Self: Film and TV Workers Report*. Singapore: Institute for Adult Learning.

Bound, H., Evans, K., Sadik, S. and Karmel, A. (2015) *How Non-Permanent Workers Learn and Develop: Challenges and Opportunities*. Singapore: Institute for Adult Learning.

Bradshaw, A. (2017) What is a nurse? The Francis Report and the historic voice of nursing. *Nursing Inquiry*, 24: e12190. https://doi.org/10.1111.nin.12190

Bradshaw, A. and Merriman, C. (2008) Nursing competence 10 years on: fit for practice and purpose yet? *Journal of Clinical Nursing*, 17: 1263–1269.

Brammer, J. D. (2006) RN as gatekeeper: student understanding of the RN buddy role in clinical practice experience. *Nurse Education Today*, 26: 697–704.

Bu, X. and Jezewski, M. A. (2007) Developing a mid-range theory of patient advocacy through concept analysis. *Journal of Advanced Nursing*, 57(1): 101–110.

Bugaj, T. J. and Nikendei, C. (2016) Practical clinical training in skills labs: Theory and practice. *GMS Journal for Medical Education*, 33(4). Retrieved from: www.ncbi.nlm.nih.gov/pmc/articles/PMC5003146/

Butterworth, T. (2014) Board editorial: the nursing profession and its leaders: hiding in plain sight? *Journal of Research in Nursing*, 19(7–8): 533–536.

Cahill, H. A. (1996) A qualitative analysis of student nurses' experiences of mentorship. *Journal of Advanced Nursing*, 24: 791–799.

Cameron, A. (2011) Impermeable boundaries? Development in professional inter-professional practice. *Journal of Interprofessional Care*, 25(1): 53–88.

Cameron, A. M., Bostock, L. and Lart, R. A. (2014) Service user and carers perspectives of joint and integrated working between health and social care. *Journal of Integrated Care*, 22(2): 62–70.

Carper, B. (1978) Fundamental patterns of knowing, *Advances in Nursing Science*, 1(1): 13–23.

Carr, W. (1986) Theories of theory and practice. *Journal of Philosophy of Education*, 20(20): 177–186.

Chinn, P. and Kramer, M. K. (1995) *Theory and Nursing: An Integrated Approach to Knowledge Development*. 5th ed. St Louis: C. V. Mosby.

Chinn, P. and Kramer, M. K. (2011) *Integrated Theory and Knowledge Development in Nursing*. 8th ed. St Louis: Elsevier, Mosby.

Chisholm, L. (2008) Re-contextualising learning in second modernity. *Research in Post-Compulsory Education*, 13(2): 139–147.

Cipriano, P. (2010) Overview and summary: delegation dilemmas: standards and skills for practice. *The Online Journal of Issues in Nursing*, 15(2). doi: 10.3912/OJIN. Vol15No02ManOS

Clouder, L. (2005) Caring as a 'threshold concept': transforming students in higher education into health(care) professionals. *Teaching in Higher Education*, 10(4): 505–517.

Cook-Sather, A. and Alter, Z. (2011) What is and what can be: how a liminal position can change learning and teaching in higher education. *Anthropology and Education Quarterly*, 42(1): 37–53.

Cooper, J., Courtney-Pratt, H. and Fitzgerald, M. (2015) Key influences identified by first year undergraduate nursing students as impacting on the quality of clinical placement: A qualitative study. *Nurse Education Today*, 35: 1004 –1008.

Cousin, G. (2006) An introduction to threshold concepts. *Planet*, No. 17(December): 4–5. Retrieved from: DOI: 10.11120/plan.2006.00170004 https://doi.org/10.11120/plan.2006.00170004

Cribb, A. and Bignold, S. (1999) Towards the reflexive medical school: the hidden curriculum and medical education research. *Studies in Higher Education*, 24: 195– 209.

Currie, G., Finn, F. and Martin, G. (2010) Role transition and the interaction of relational and social identity: new nursing roles in the English NHS. *Organization Studies*, 31(7): 941–961.

Dahlgren, G. and Whitehead, M. (2007 [1993]) Tackling inequalities in health: what can we learn from what has been tried? Working paper prepared for the King's Fund International Seminar on Tackling Inequalities in Health, September 1993, Ditchley Park, Oxfordshire. London, King's Fund. In D. Goran and M. Whitehead (eds), *European Strategies for Tackling Social Inequities in Health: Levelling up Part 2*. Copenhagen: WHO Regional office for Europe. Retrieved from: www.euro.who.int/__data/assets/pdf_file/0018/103824/E89384.pdf

Davies, C. (1995) *Gender and the Professional Predicament of Nursing*. Buckingham: Open University Press.

Davies, C. (2003) Some of our concepts are missing: reflections on the absence of a sociology of organizations. *Sociology of Health and Illness*, 25 (Silver Anniversary Issue): 172–190.

Davies, C. (2004) Regulating the health care workforce: next steps for research. *Journal of Health Services Research & Policy*, 9(Suppl 1): 55–61.

Davies, C., Anand, P., Artigas, L., Holloway, J., McConway, K., Newman, J., Storey, J. and Thompson, G. (2005) *Links between Governance, Incentives and Outcomes: a Review of the Literature*. Report for the National Co-ordinating Centre for NHS Service Delivery and Organisation R & D (NCCSDO). London: NCCSDO

Department of Health (1995) *Patient's Charter*. London: HMSO.

Department of Health (1999) *Making a Difference: Strengthening the Nursing, Midwifery and Health Visiting Contribution to Health and Healthcare*. London: HMSO.

Department of Health (2000) *NHS Plan*. London: HMSO.

Department of Health (2001) *The Expert Patient: A New Approach to Chronic Disease in the 21st century*. London: HMSO.

Department of Health (2011) *Government Response to the NHS Future Forum Report*. London: HMSO.

Department of Health (2012) *The Health & Social Care Act*. London: HMSO.

Department of Health (2013) *Delivering High Quality, Effective, Compassionate Care: Developing the Right People with the Right Skills and the Right Values. A Mandate from the Government to Health Education England*. London: HMSO.

Dewey, J. (1933) *How We Think*. Boston: D.C. Heath.

Dewing, J. (2008) Becoming and being active learners and creating active learning workplaces: the value of active learning in practice development. In K. Manley, B. McCormack and V. Wilson (eds), *International Practice Development in Nursing and Healthcare*. Oxford: Blackwell. pp. 273–294.

Dickoff, J. and James, P. (1968) A theory of theories: a position paper. *Nursing Research*, 17(3): 197–203.

Donaldson, S. K. and Crowley, D. M. (1978) The discipline of nursing. *Nursing Outlook*, 26(2): 113–120.

Drevdahl, D. and Canales, M. (2020) Being a real nurse: a secondary qualitative analysis of how public health nurses rework their work identities. *Nursing Inquiry*, 27(4): e12360.

Ehrenreich, B. and English, D. (1979) *For Her Own Good: 100 Years of Advice to Women*. London: Pluto Press.

Emirbayer, M. and Mische, A. (1998). What is agency? *American Journal of Sociology*, 103(4): 962–1023.

Eraut, M. (1994) *Developing Professional Knowledge and Competence*. London: Routledge, Falmer Press.

Eraut, M. (2000) Non-formal learning and tacit knowledge in professional work. *British Journal of Educational Psychology*, 70: 113–136.

Eraut, M., Alderton, J., Boylan, A. and Wraight, A. (1995) *Learning to use Scientific Knowledge in Education and Practice Settings*. London: English National Board for Nursing, Midwifery and Health Visiting.

Eraut, M., Alderton, J., Boylan, A. and Wraight, A. (1996) Mediating scientific knowledge into health care practice: Evidence from pre-registration programmes in nursing and midwifery education. Paper presented at AERA Conference, New York, April 1996.

Evans, K. (2015) Developing knowledgeable practice at work. In M. Elg, P.-E. Ellstrom, M. Klofsten and M. Tillmar (eds), *Sustainable Development in Organizations Studies on Innovative Practices*. Cheltenham: Edward Elgar. pp. 109–126.

Evans, K. (2017) Bounded agency in professional lives. In M. Goller and S. Paloniemi (eds), *Agency at Work. Professional and Practice-based Learning*, Vol. 20. New York: Springer. pp. 1–26.

Evans, K. (2020) Learning ecologies at work. In R. Barnett and N. Jackson (eds), *Ecologies for Learning and Practice*. London: Routledge. pp. 163–176.

Evans, K. and Guile, D. (2012) Putting different forms of knowledge to work in practice. In J. Higgs, S. Billett, M. Hutchings and F. Trede (eds), *Practice-Based Education: Perspectives and Strategies*. Rotterdam: Sense Publishers. pp. 113 –136.

Evans, K., Kersh, N. and Kontiainen, S. (2004) Recognition of tacit skills: sustaining learning outcomes in adult learning and work re-entry. *International Journal of Training and Development*, 8: 54–72.

Evans, K., Hodkinson, P., Rainbird, H. and Unwin, L. (2006) *Improving Workplace Learning*. Abingdon: Routledge.

Evans, K., Guile, D. and Harris, J. (2009) *Putting Knowledge to Work: The Exemplars. Centre for Excellence in Work-Based Learning (WLE Centre) UCL Institute of Education*. London: University of London.

Evans, K., Guile, D., Harris, J. and Allan, H. T. (2010) Putting knowledge to work: a new approach. *Nurse Education Today*, 30: 245–251.

Evans, M. (2009) Tackling the theory–practice gap in mental health nurse training. *Mental Health Practice*, 13(2): 21–24.

Evans, W. and Kelly, W. (2004) Pre-registration diploma student nurse stress and coping measures. *Nurse Education Today*, 24: 473–482.

Eveleigh, M. (2018) Safe delegation techniques for practice nurses. *Nursing in Practice*. Retrieved from: www.nursinginpractice.com/safe-delegation-techniques-practice-nurses (accessed 15 November 2019).

Fabricius, J. (1991) Running on the spot or can nursing really change. *Psychoanalytic Psychotherapy*, 5: 97–108.

Fabricius, J. (1995) Psychoanalytic understanding and nursing: a supervisory workshop with nurse tutors. *Psychoanalytic Psychotherapy*, 9:17–29.

Fabricius, J. (1999) The crisis in nursing: reflections on the crisis. *Psychoanalytic Psychotherapy*, 13(3): 203–206.

Fairman, J. (1997) Thinking about patients: nursing science in the 1950s. *Reflections*, 23: 30–32.

Fairman, J. (2008) Context and contingency in the history of post World War II nursing scholarship in the United States. *Journal of Nursing Scholarship*, 40(1): 4–11.

Fawcett, J. (1992) Contemporary conceptualisations of nursing: philosophy or science? In J. F. Kikuchi and H. Simmons (eds), *Philosophic Inquiry in Nursing*. Newbury Park, CA: Sage. pp. 64–70.

Fawcett, J. (2005) *Contemporary Nursing Knowledge: Analysis and Evaluation of Nursing models and Theories*. 2nd ed. Philadelphia: F.A. Davis.

Fealy, G. M. (1999) The theory-practice relationship in nursing: the practitioner's perspective. *Journal of Advanced Nursing*, 30(1): 72–82.

Field, D. (2004) Moving from novice to expert – the value of learning in clinical practice: a literature review. *Nurse Education Today*, 24: 560–565.

Fitzpatrick, J. J. and Whall, A. L. (1996) *Conceptual Models of Nursing: Analysis and Application*. 3rd ed. St Louis: C. V. Mosby.

Forber, J., DiGiacomo, M., Davidson, P., Carter, B. and Jackson, D. (2015) The context, influences and challenges for undergraduate nurse clinical education: continuing the dialogue. *Nurse Education Today*, 35: 1114–1118.

Forsman, H., Rudman, A., Gustavsson, P., Ehrenberg, A. and Wallin, L. (2012) Nurses' research utilization two years after graduation: a national survey of associated individual, organizational, and educational factors. *Implementation Science*, 7(46): 1–12.

Francis, R. (2013) *Report of the Mid Staffordshire NHS Foundation Trust Public Inquiry: Robert Francis QC (Chair)*. HC 898 1–111. London: HMSO.

Francisco, S. (2020) Developing a trellis of practices that support learning in the workplace. *Studies in Continuing Education*, 42(1): 102 –117.

Franklin, B. (2014) *The Future Care Workforce*. London: Anchor, ILC-UK. Retrieved from: https:ilcuk.org.uk

Freshwater, D. and Rolfe, G. (2001) Critical reflexivity: a politically and ethically engaged research method for nursing. *NT Research*, 6: 526–537.

Gallagher, P. (2004) How the metaphor of a gap between theory and practice has influenced nursing education. *Nurse Education Today*, 24(4): 263–268.

Gerrish, K. (2001) A pluralistic evaluation of nursing/practice development units. *Journal of Clinical Nursing*, 10(1): 109–118.

Gill, D. (2013) *Becoming doctors: The formation of professional identity in newly qualified doctors*. Doctoral thesis, UCL Institute of Education. Retrieved from: https://discovery.ucl.ac.uk/id/eprint/10020735/

Glasby, J. (2006) We have to stop meeting like this: The governance of inter-agency partnerships. A discussion article. University of Birmingham, Health Services Management Centre, Institute of Local Government Studies. Retrieved from: www.icn.csip.org.uk

Glasby, J. and Dickinson, H. (2008) *Partnership Working in Health and Social Care*. Bristol: Policy Press/Community Care.

Glasby, J., Martin, G. and Regen, E. (2008) Older people and the relationship between hospital services and intermediate care: results from a national evaluation. *Journal of Interprofessional Care*, 2(6): 639–649.

Goodrich, J. and Cornwall, J. (2008) *Seeing The Person in The Patient: The Point of Care Review Paper*. London: The King's Fund.

Gramling, K. L. (2004) A narrative study of nursing art in critical care. *Journal of Holistic Nursing*, 22(4): 379–398.

Grant, J. and Guerin, P. C. (2018) Mixed and misunderstandings: an exploration of the meaning of racism with maternal, child, and family health nurses in South Australia. *Journal of Advanced Nursing*, 74(12): 2831–2839.

Gravlin, G. and Bittner, N. P. (2010) Nurses' and nursing assistants' reports of missed care and delegation. *Journal of Nursing Administration*, 40(7–8): 329–335.

Gray, A. (2016) Advanced or advancing nursing practice: what is the future direction for nursing? *British Journal Nursing*, 25(1): 8, 10, 12–13.

Greenberg, N. and Rafferty, L. (2021) Post-traumatic stress disorder in the aftermath of COVID-19 pandemic. *World Psychiatry*, 20(1): 53–54.

Groothuizen, J. E., Callwood, A. and Allan, H. T. (2019) The 'values journey' of nursing and midwifery students selected using multiple mini interviews: evaluations from a longitudinal study. *Nursing Inquiry*, 26(4): e12307.

Guile, D. and Evans, K. (2010) *Putting Knowledge to Work: Re-contextualising Knowledge through the Design and Implementation of Work-based Learning at Higher Education Levels.* Retrieved from: https://s3.eu-west-2.amazonaws.com/assets.creode.advancehe-document-manager/documents/hea/private/putting-knowledge-to-work_1568037385.pdf

Hall, P. (2005) Interprofessional teamwork: professional cultures as barriers. *Journal of Interprofessional Care*, 19(5): 188–196.

Harding Clark, S. C. (2006) *The Lourdes Hospital Inquiry: An Inquiry into Peripartum Hysterectomy at Our Lady of Lourdes Hospital, Drogheda.* Dublin: TSO.

Haskvitz, L. M. and Koop, E. C. (2004) Students struggling in clinical? A new role for the patient simulator. *The Journal of Nursing Education*, 43(4): 181–184.

Hasson, F., McKenna, H. P. and Keeney, S. (2013) Delegating and supervising unregistered professionals: the student nurse experience. *Nurse Education Today*, 33(3): 229–235.

Hazell, W. (2015) Worcestershire trust's bullying policy 'not fit for purpose'. *Health Service Journal*, 27 August.

Health Education England/Nursing and Midwifery Council (2015) *Raising the Bar Shape of Caring: A Review of the Future Education and Training of Registered Nurses and Care Assistants Lord Willis, Independent Chair – Shape of Caring Review.* Retrieved from: www.hee.nhs.uk/sites/default/files/documents/2348-Shape-of-caring-review-FINAL.pdf

Heggen, K. (2008) Social workers, teachers and nurses – from college to professional work. *Journal of Education and Work*, 21(3): 217–231.

Henderson, V. (1966) *The Nature of Nursing: A Definition and its Implications for Practice.* New York: Macmillan.

Henderson, V. (1991) *The Nature of Nursing: Reflections after 25 Years.* New York: National League of Nursing Press.

Hinchcliffe, G. (2013) Workplace identity, transition and the role of learning. In P. Gibbs (ed.), *Learning Work and Practice: New Understandings.* Dordrecht: Springer. pp. 51–69.

Hökkä, P. K., Vähäsantanen, K., Paloniemi, S. and Eteläpelto, A. (2017) The reciprocal relationship between emotions and agency in the workplace. In M. Goller and S. Paloniemi (eds), *Professional and Practice-based Learning: Vol. 20. Agency at Work: An Agentic Perspective on Professional Learning and Development.* Cham: Springer. pp. 161–181.

Holder, H., Robertson, R., Ross, S., Bennett, L., Gosling, J. and Curry, N. (2015) *Risk or Reward: The Changing Role of CCGs in General Practice. Research Report.* London: The King's Fund and Nuffield Trust.

Holland, D., Lachicotte, W. Jr, Skinner, D. and Cain, C. (1998) *Identity and Agency in Cultural Worlds.* Cambridge, MA: Harvard University Press.

House of Commons Health Committee (2017–2019) *The Nursing Workforce Second Report of Session HC353.* Retrieved from: https://publications.parliament.uk/pa/cm201719/cmselect/cmhealth/353/353.pdf (accessed 15 November 2019).

Imison, C., Castle-Clarke, S. and Watson, R. (2016). Reshaping the workforce to deliver the care patients need. Retrieved from: www.nuffieldtrust.org.uk/research/reshaping-the-workforce-to-deliver-the-care-patients-need

International Council of Nursing (2002) Nursing definitions. Retrieved from: www.icn.ch/nursing-policy/nursing-definitions

Jackson, C. and Thurgate, C. (eds) (2011) *Workplace Learning in Health and Social Care: A Student's Guide*. Maidenhead: Open University Press.

Jackson, D. and Mannix, J. (2001) Clinical nurses as teachers: insights from students of nursing in their first semester of study. *Journal of Clinical Nursing*, 10(2): 270–277.

Jackson, D., Hutchinson, M., Peters, K. and Luck, L. (2012) Understanding avoidant leadership in healthcare: findings from a secondary analysis of two qualitative studies. *Journal of Nursing Management*, 21: 572–580.

Jackson, N. and Barnett, R. (2020) Steps to ecologies for learning and practice. In R. Barnett and N. Jackson (eds), *Ecologies for Learning and Practice: Emerging Ideas, Sightings and Possibilities*. Abingdon: Routledge. pp. 1–16.

Jacobs, M. (1991) *Psychodynamic Counselling in Action*. London: Sage.

James, A. and Chapman, Y. (Dec 2009/Jan 2010) Preceptors and patients – the power of two: nursing student experiences on their first acute clinical placement. *Contemporary Nurse*, 34(1): 34–47.

Jeffries, P., Rew, S. and Cramer, J. (2002) A comparison of student centered versus traditional methods of teaching basic nursing skills in a learning laboratory. *Nursing Education Perspectives*, 23: 14–19.

Jensen, K. and Lahn, L. (2005) The binding role of knowledge: an analysis of nursing students' knowledge ties. *Journal of Education and Work*, 18: 305–320.

Johnson, M., Magnusson, C., Allan, H. T., Evans, K., Ball, E. and Horton, K. (2015) Doing the writing and working in parallel: how 'distal nursing' affects delegation and supervision in the emerging role of the newly qualified nurse. Special Edition. *Nurse Education Today*, 35(2): e29–33. doi.org/10.1016/j.nedt.2014.11.020

Jones, A. and Kelly, D. (2014) Whistleblowing and workplace culture in older people's care: insights form the healthcare and social care workforce. *Sociology of Health & Illness*, 36: 986–1002.

Kaur, S., Radford, M. and Arblaster, G. (2016) A framework for advanced clinical practice. *Nursing Times*, 112(19): 22–24.

Kermode, S. and Brown, C. (2011) The postmodernist hoax and its effects on nursing. *International Journal of Nursing Studies*, 33(4): 375–384.

Kersh, K., Waite, E. and Evans, K. (2011a) *The Spatial Dimensions of Skills for Life Workplace Provision, Institute of Education*. London: Centre for Learning and Life Chances in Knowledge Economies and Societies. Retrieved from: www.llakes.ac.uk/sites/default/files/24.%20Kersh%20Waite%20Evans%20-%20final.pdf (accessed 6 December 2019).

Kersh, N., Evans, K., Kontianinen, S. and Bailey, H. (2011b) Use of conceptual models in self-evaluation of personal competences in learning and planning for change. *International Journal of Training and Development*, 15(4): 290–305.

Kikuchi, J. F. and Simmons, H. (eds) (1992) *Philosophic Inquiry in Nursing*. Thousand Oaks, CA: Sage.

Kira, M. (2010) Routine-generating and regenerative workplace learning. *Vocations and Learning*, 3(1): 71–90.

Kirpal, M. and Simone, R. (2004) Work identities of nurses: between caring and efficiency demands. *Career Development International*, 9: 274–304.

Kitson, A. (2002) Recognising relationships: reflections on evidence-based practice. *Nursing Inquiry*, 9(3): 179–186.

Kolcaba, K. (2003) *A Comfort Theory and Practice: A Vision for Holistic Health Care and Research*. New York: Springer.

Kong, B.-Y. (2004) Post modernism and the issue of nursing. *Journal of Korean Academy of Nursing*, 34(3): 389–399.

Laiho, A. and Ruoholinna, T. (2013) The relationship between practitioners and academics – anti-academic discourse voiced by Finnish nurses. *Journal of Vocational Education and Training*, 65(3): 333–350.

Lambert, N. (2021) Building a community of digital professional practice. Presentation to Scholars at Work Seminar, Middlesex University.

Land, R., Cousin, G., Meyer, J. H. F. and Davies, P. (2005) Threshold concepts and troublesome knowledge (3): implications for course design and evaluation. In C. Rust (ed.), *Improving Student Learning Diversity and Inclusivity*. Oxford: Oxford Centre for Staff and Learning Development. pp. 53–64.

Land, R., Meyer, J. H. F. and Baillie, C. (2010) Editors' preface: threshold concepts and transformational learning. In R. Land, J. H. F., Meyer and C. Baillie (eds), *Threshold Concepts and Transformational Learning*. Rotterdam: Sense Publishers. pp. ix–xiii.

Land, R., Rattray, J., Vivian, P. and Ashwin, P. (2014) Learning in the liminal space: a semiotic approach to threshold concepts. *Higher Education*, 67(2): 199–217.

Lapum, J., Fredericks, S., Beanlands, H., McCay, E., Schwind, J. and Romaniuk, D. (2012) A cyborg ontology in health care: traversing into the liminal space between technology and person-centred practice. *Nursing Philosophy*, 13(4): 276–288.

Larbi, G. A. (1999) The new public management approach and crisis states. Retrieved from: www.unrisd.org/80256B3C005BCCF9/(httpPublications)/5F280B19C6125F4380256B66 00448FDB (accessed 15 November 2019).

Latimer, J. (2014) Guest editorial: Nursing and the politics of organisation and the meanings of care. *Journal of Nursing Research*, 19(7–8): 537–545.

Lave, J. and Wenger, E. (1991) *Learning in doing: Social, cognitive, and computational perspectives. Situated learning: Legitimate peripheral participation*. Cambridge: Cambridge University Press.

Lawler, J. (1991) *Behind the Screens: Nursing, Somology and the Problem of the Body*. Australia; University of Sydney: Churchill Livingstone.

Lawler, J. A. (2005) Leadership in social work: a case of caveat emptor. *British Journal of Social Work*, 37(1): 123–141.

Leininger, M. (1981) *Caring: An Essential Human Need*. Thorofare, NJ: Slack.

Leininger, M. (2002) *Transcultural Nursing: Concepts, Theories, Research and Practice*. New York: McGraw-Hill.

Lemke, J. L. (2000) Across the scales of time: artifacts, activities and meanings in ecosocial systems. *Mind, Culture and Activity*, 7(4): 273–290.

LeVasseur, J. (1999) Towards an understanding of art in nursing. *Advances in Nursing Science*, 21(4): 48–63.

Levett-Jones, T., Lathlean, J., Higgins, I. and McMillan, M. (2009) The duration of clinical placements: a key influence on nursing students' experience of belongingness. *Australian Journal of Advanced Nursing* (Online), 26(2): 8–16.

Loo, S. (2014) Placing 'knowledge' in teacher education in the English further education sector: an alternative approach based on collaboration and evidence-based research. *British Journal of Educational Studies*, 62(3): 337–354.

Mackintosh, M. (1992) Partnership: issues of policy and negotiation. *Local Economy*, 7(3): 210–224.

Maclaine, K. (2017) Steps towards an advanced clinical practice standard. *Nursing Management*, 24(1): 18.

Magnusson, C., Allan, H. T., Horton, K., Johnson, M., Evans, K. and Ball, E. (2017) An analysis of delegation styles among newly qualified nurses. *Nursing Standard*, 31(25): 46–53.

Manley, K. (1997) Knowledge for nursing practice. In A. Perry (ed.), *Nursing a Knowledge Base for Practice*. 2nd ed. London: Arnold. pp. 301–330.

Manley, K. and Webster, J. (2006) Can we keep quality care alive? *Nursing Standard*, 21(3): 12–15.

Manley, K., Titchen, A. and Hardy, S. (2009) Work based learning in the context of contemporary healthcare education and practice: a concept analysis. *Practice Development in Health Care*, (8)2: 87–127.

Manley, K., Hils, V. and Marriot, S. (2011) Person-centred care: Principle of Nursing Practice

D. *Nursing Standard*, 25(31): 35–37.

Manley, K., O'Keefe, H., Jackson, C., Pearce, J. and Smith, S. (2014) A shared purpose framework to deliver person-centred, safe and effective care: organisational transformation using practice development methodology. *International Practice Development Journal*, 4(1): 1–28.

Marmot, M., Allen, J., Goldblatt, P., Boyce, T., McNeish, D., Grady, M. and Geddes, I. (2010) *Fair Society, Healthy Lives. The Health Foundation and the Institute of Health Inequity*. Retrieved from: www.instituteofhealthequity.org/resources-reports/fair-society-healthy-lives-the-marmot-review (accessed 12 July 2019).

Marmot, M., Allen, J., Boyce, T., Goldblatt, P. and Morrison, J. (2020) *Health Equity in England: The Marmot Review 10 Years On. The Health Foundation and the Institute of Health Inequity*. Retrieved from: www.health.org.uk/publications/reports/the-marmot-review-10-years-on

May, C., Eton, D. T., Boehmer, K., Gallacher, K., Hunt, K., MacDonald, S., Mair, F. S., May, C. M., Montori, V. M., Richardson, A., Rogers, A. E. and Shipee, N. (2014) Rethinking the patient: using Burden of Treatment Theory to understand the changing dynamics of illness. *BMC Health Services Research*, 14: 288.

McBride, A. B. (1996) Professional nursing education: today and tomorrow. In S. G. Wunderlich, F. Sloan and C. K. Davies (eds), *Nursing Staff in Hospitals and Nursing Homes: Is it Adequate?* Washington, DC: National Academic Press. pp. 333–360.

McCann, S., Olphert, A. M. and Minogue, V. (2014) The role of the CCG nurse in commissioning services. *Nursing Times*, 110(48): 15–17.

McCormack, B. and McCance, T. (2010) *Person-centred Nursing: Theory and Practice*. Oxford: Wiley-Blackwell.

McCormack, B., Manley, K. and Walsh, K. (2008) Person-centred systems and processes. In K. Manley, B. McCormack and V. J. Wilson (eds), *International Practice Development in Nursing and Healthcare*. Oxford: Wiley-Blackwell. pp. 17–41.

McCrae, N. (2012) Whither nursing models? The value of nursing theory in the context of evidence-based practice and multidisciplinary health care. *Journal of Advanced Nursing*, 68(1): 222–229.

McKenna, H. (1997) *Nursing Theories and Models*. London: Routledge.

McKenna, H. and Slevin, O. D. (2008) *Nursing Models: Theories and Practice*. Oxford: Blackwell.

McMahon, M. and Kimberley, C. (2011) Toward a mid-range theory of nursing presence. *Nursing Forum*, 46(2): 71–82.

Meijers, J. M. M., Janssen, M. E. I., Jers, J .M., Cummings, G. G., Wallin, L., Estabrooks, C. A. and Halfens, R. Y. G. (2006) Assessing the relationships between contextual factors and research utilization in nursing: systematic literature review. *Journal of Advanced Nursing*, 55(5): 622–635.

Meleis, A. I. (1991) *Theoretical Nursing: Development and Progress*. 2nd ed. Philidelphia: Lippincott.

Meleis, A. (1992) Directions for nursing theory developments in the 21st century. In F. Murphy and C. Smith (eds), *Nursing Theories and Models*, Vol. 3:47–258. London: Sage Publications.

Melia, K. (2006) R000271191 – Nursing in the new NHS: a sociological analysis of learning and working.

Menzies-Lyth, I. E. P. (1970) *The Functioning of Social Systems as a Defence Against Anxiety: Report on a Study of the Nursing Service of a General Hospital*. London: The Tavistock Institute of Human Relations.

Merriam, S. B. and Caffarella, R. S. (1999) *Learning in Adulthood: A Comprehensive Guide*. San Francisco, CA: Jossey-Bass.

Miller, A. E. (1989) The relationship between nursing theory and nursing practice. In M. Jolley and P. Allan (eds), *Current Issues in Nursing*. London: Chapman Hall. pp. 47–66.

Morgan, R. (2006) Using clinical skills laboratories to promote theory–practice integration during first practice placement: an Irish perspective. *Journal of Clinical Nursing*, 15: 155–161.

Mothers and Babies: Reducing Risk through Audits and Confidential Enquiries across the UK (MBRRACE-UK) (2018) *Saving Lives, Improving Mothers' Care: Reducing Risk through Audits and Confidential Enquiries across the UK*. Retrieved from: www.npeu.ox.ac.uk/downloads/files/mbrrace-uk/reports/MBRRACE-UK%20Maternal%20Report%20 2018%20-%20Web%20Version.pdf

Muls, A., Dougherty, L., Doyle, N., Shaw, C., Soanes, L. and Stevens, A. M. (2015) Influencing organisational culture: a leadership challenge. *British Journal of Nursing*, 24(12): 633–638.

Murphy, F; and Smith, C. (2013) *Nursing Theories and Models*. Vols 1–3. London: Sage.

Neumann, T. A. (2010) Delegation – better safe than sorry. *AAOHN* (American Association of Occupational Health Nurses), 58(8): 321–322.

Newton, J. N. et al. (2015) Changes in health in England, with analysis by English regions and areas of deprivation, 1990–2013: a systematic analysis for the Global Burden of Disease Study. *The Lancet*, 386(10010): 2257–2274.

NHS (2018) Workforce statistics – including supplementary analysis on pay by ethnicity. Retrieved from: https://digital.nhs.uk/data-and-information/publications/statistical/nhs-workforce-statistics/june-2018

NHS (2019) The long term plan. Retrieved from: www.england.nhs.uk/long-term-plan/

NHS Commissioning Board (2012) Clinical commissioning group governing body members: Role outlines, attributes and skills. Retrieved from: www.england.nhs.uk/wp-content/uploads/2016/09/ccg-members-roles.pdf

NHS England (2012) *The 'Right People, with the Right Skills, are in the Right Place at the Right Time'? A Guide to Nursing, Midwifery, and Care Staffing Capacity and Capability*. Retrieved from: www.england.nhs.uk/wp-content/uploads/2013/11/nqb-how-to-guid.pdf

NHS England (2014) *Winterbourne View – Time for Change. Transforming the Commissioning of Services for People with Learning Disability and Autism. A Report by the Transforming Care and Commissioning Group, chaired by Sir Stephen Bubb*. Retrieved from: www.england.nhs.uk/wp-content/uploads/2014/11/transforming-commissioning-services.pdf

NHS England (2016a) *Compassion in Practice – Evidencing the Impact*. Retrieved from: www.england.nhs.uk/wp-content/uploads/2016/05/CiPVS-yr-3.pdf

NHS England (2016b) *Leading Change, Adding Value: A Framework for Nursing, Midwifery and Care Staff*. Retrieved from: www.england.nhs.uk/wp-content/uploads/2016/05/nursing-framework.pdf

NHS Executive (2012) *Compassion in Practice. Nursing, Midwifery and Care Staff. Our Vision and Strategy*. Leeds: Department of Health and NHS Commissioning Board.

NHS Improvement (2019) *Gender Pay Gap Report 2017 to 2018*. Retrieved from: www.england.nhs.uk/wp-content/uploads/2018/03/gender-pay-gap-report-march-2019.pdf (accessed 12 July 2019).

Nieminen, P. (2008) Caught in the science trap? A case study of the relationship between nurses and 'their' science. In J. Välimaa and O.-H. Ylijoki (eds), *Cultural Perspectives on Higher Education*. New York: Springer. pp. 127–141.

NMC (2013) *Response to the Francis Report. The Response of the Nursing and Midwifery Council to the Mid Staffordshire NHS Foundation Trust Public Inquiry Report*. Retrieved from: www.nmc.org.uk/globalassets/sitedocuments/francis-report/nmc-response-to-the-francis-report-18-july.pdf (accessed 24 July 2019).

NMC (2018a) *Future Nurse: Standards of Proficiency for Registered Nurses*. Retrieved from: www.nmc.org.uk/globalassets/sitedocuments/education-standards/future-nurse-proficiencies.pdf

NMC (2018b) *Standards Framework for Nursing and Midwifery Education*. Retrieved from: www.nmc.org.uk/standards-for-education-and-training/

O'Driscoll, M., Allan, H. T. and Smith, P. (2010) Still looking for leadership – who is responsible for students nurses' learning in practice? *Nurse Education Today*, 30(3): 212–218.

O'Driscoll, M., Allan, H. T., Serrant, L., Corbett, K. and Lui, L. (2018a) Compassion in practice

– evaluating the awareness, involvement and perceived impact of a national nursing and midwifery strategy amongst health care professionals in NHS Trusts in England. *Journal of Clinical Nursing*, 27(5–6): e1097–e1109. doi: 10.1111/jocn.14176

O'Driscoll, M., Allan, H. T., Savage, J., Lee, G. and Dixon, R. (2018b) Do Governing Body and CSU nurses on Clinical Commissioning Groups really lead a nursing agenda? *Journal of Nursing Management*, 26(3): 245–255.

O'Shea, A., Chambers, M. and Boaz, A. (2013) Whose voices? Patient and public involvement in clinical commissioning. *Health Expectations*, 20(3): 484–494.

O'Toole, L., Hayes, N. and Halpenny, A. M. (2020) Animating systems: the ecological value of Bronfenbrenner's bioecological model of development. In R. Barnett and N. Jackson (eds), *Ecologies for learning and Practice: Emerging Ideas, Sightings and Possibilities*. Abingdon: Routledge. pp. 19–31.

Oakley, A. (1986) On the importance of being a nurse. In A. Oakley (ed.), *Telling the Truth about the New Jerusalem: A Collection of Essays and Poems*. Oxford: Blackwell. pp. 180–195.

Paley, J. (2014) Cognition and the compassion deficit: the social psychology of helping behaviour in nursing. *Nursing Philosophy*, 15(4): 274–287.

Pawson, R. and Tilley, N. (2004) *Realist evaluation*. London: Sage Publication.

Pearcey, P. A. and Elliott, B. E. (2004) Student impressions of clinical nursing. *Nurse Education Today*, 24(5): 382–387.

Peplau, H. (1988) *Interpersonal Relations in Nursing*. Basingstoke: Macmillan Education.

Porter, S. (1995) *Nursing's Relationship with Medicine*. Aldershot: Avebury.

Porter, S. (1998) *Social Theory and Nursing Practice*. London: Macmillan.

Poulton, B. and West, M. (1999) The determinants of effectiveness in primary health care teams. *Journal of Interprofessional Care*, 13(1): 7–18.

Public Health England (2017) The social determinants of health. In: *Health Profile for England: 2017 A Report Combining Data and Knowledge with Information from Other Sources to Give a Broad Picture of the Health of People in England in 2017*. Retrieved from: www.gov.uk/government/publications/health-profile-for-england/chapter-6-social-determinants-of-health

Public Health England (2018) London Knowledge and Intelligence Team: Protecting and improving the nation's health. Retrieved from: https://assets.publishing.service.gov.uk/government/uploads/system/uploads/attachment_data/file/730917/local_action_on_health_inequalities.pdf (accessed 23 July 2019).

Purkis, M. E. and Bjornsdottir, K. (2006) Intelligent nursing: accounting for knowledge as action. *Nursing Philosophy*, 7(4): 247–256.

Quinlan, K. and Song, Y. (1998) Cognitive theory: its implications for vocational education and training. *Canadian Vocational Journal*, 33(3): 5–8.

RCN (1985a) *The Education of Nurses: A New Dispensation. Commission on Nursing Education. Chairman, Dr. Harry Judge*. London: RCN.

RCN (1985b) *Annexe of Research Studies for Commission on Nursing Education, The Education of Nurses: A New Dispensation*. London: RCN.

RCN (2012) Nurse membership on clinical commissioning group governing bodies. Royal College of Nursing. Retrieved from: file:///C:/Users/Helen54/History/IE/6Q9ZTH4Q/1912.pdf (accessed 4 March 2015).

RCN (2017) *Accountability and Delegation: A Guide for the Nursing Team*. London: RCN.

RCN (2018a) RCN Response to the Health Education England (HEE) consultation on Facing the Facts, Shaping the Future – a draft health and care workforce strategy for England to 2017. Retrieved from: file:///C:/Users/Helen54/History/IE/0VJESAMX/CONR-5817.pdf (accessed 15 November 2019).

RCN (2018b) *An RCN Education and Career Progression Framework for Fertility Nursing*. Retrieved from: https://www.rcn.org.uk/professional-development/publications/pdf-006690 (accessed 8 November 2019).

Read, S., Jones, M., Collins, K., McDonnell, A., Jones, R., Doyal, L., Cameron, A., Masterson,

A., Dowling, S., Vaughan, B., Furlong, A. and Scholes, J. (2001) *Exploring New Roles in Practice (ENRiP) Final Report*. Sheffield: University of Sheffield, ScHARR.

Rebeiro, G., Edward, K.-L., Chapman, R. and Evans, A. (2015) Interpersonal relationships between registered nurses and student nurses in the clinical setting: a systematic integrative review. *Nurse Education Today*, 35(12): 1206–1211.

Reed, P. G. (2006a) A treatise on nursing knowledge development for the 21st century: beyond postmodernism. In F. Murphy and C. Smith (eds), *Nursing Theories and Models*. Vol. 3. London: Sage. pp. 27–44.

Reed, P. G. (2006b) Commentary on neomodernism and evidence-based nursing: implications for the production of nursing knowledge. *Nursing Outlook*, 54: 36–38.

Rhyl, G. (1963) *The Concept of the Mind*. London: Penguin.

Richardson, B. (1999) Professional development: professional socialisation and professionalization. *Physiotherapy*, 85(9): 461–467.

Ricketts, B., Merriman, C. and Stayt, C. (2013) Simulated practice learning in a preregistration programme. *British Journal of Nursing*, 21(7): 435–440.

Roberts, D. J. (2013) The Francis report on the Mid-Staffordshire NHS Foundation Trust: putting patients first. *Transfusion Medicine*, 23(2): 73–76.

Rogers, B. (2020) *The Mountaintop and the Swamp; The Role of Time in the Practising of Change Commitments after a Customised Executive Education Programme*. Cambridge: University of Cambridge.

Rolfe, G. (1993) Closing the theory – practice gap: a model of nursing praxis. *Journal of Clinical Nursing*, 2 (3): 173–177.

Rolfe, G. (1999) The pleasure of the bottomless: postmodernism, chaos and paradigm shifts. *Nurse Education Today*, 19(8): 668–672.

Rolfe, G. (2001) Postmodernism for healthcare workers in 13 easy steps. *Nurse Education Today*, 21: 38–47.

Rolfe, G. (2005) The deconstructing angel: nursing, reflection and evidence-based practice. *Nursing Inquiry*, 12(2): 78–86.

Rolfe, G. (2006a) Nursing praxis and the science of the unique. In F. Murphy and C. Smith (eds), *Nursing Theories and Models*. Vol. 3. London: Sage. pp. 227–238.

Rolfe, G, (2006b) Review: a critical realist rationale for using a combination of quantitative and qualitative methods. *Journal of Research in Nursing*, 11(1): 79–80.

Rolfe, G. (2014) Rethinking reflective education: what would Dewey have done? *Nurse Education Today*, 34: 1179–1183.

Roper, N., Logan, W. and Tierney, A. (1985) *The Elements of Nursing*. 2nd ed. Edinburgh: Churchill Livingstone.

Ross, F., Allan, H. T., Byng, R., Christian, S., Smith, P. and Brearley, S. (2014) Learning from people with long-term conditions: understanding the professional experience of changing. *Journal of Health and Social Care in the Community*, 22(4): 405–416.

Ross, F., Christian, S., Clayton, J., Byng, R., Price, L., Smith, P., Allan, H., Redfern, S., Brearley, S., Manthorpe, J. and MacKintosh, M. M. (2009) *The Professional Experience of Governance and Incentives: Meeting the Needs of Individuals with Complex Conditions in Primary Care*. Retrieved from: file:///C:/Users/Helen54/History/IE/ZIEUCRXR/3027274.pdf (accessed 8 November 2019).

Rudge, T. (2015) Managerialism, governmentality and the evolving regulatory climate. *Nursing Inquiry*, 22(1): 1–2.

Rutter, L. (2009) 'Theory' and 'practice' within HE professional education courses – integration of academic knowledge and experiential knowledge. Presented at the 6th LDHEN Symposium: Bournemouth University, 'The Challenge of Learning Development' 6 and 7 April 2009. Retrieved from: https://core.ac.uk/download/pdf/75468.pdf

Saltman, R. B. (2003) The melting public–private boundary in European health care systems. *European Journal of Public Health*, 13(1): 24–29.

Saltman, R. B. and Figueras, J. (1997) *European Health Care Reform: Analysis of Current*

Strategies. Copenhagen: WHO Regional Office for Europe.

Sandelowski, M. (2000) *Devices and Desires: Gender, Technology and American Nursing*. New York: Springer.

Sanders, S. and Welk, D. S. (2005) Strategies to scaffold student learning applying Vygotsky's zone of proximal development. *Nurse Educator*, 30(5): 203–207.

Savin-Baden, M. (2020) Learning ecologies, liminal states and student transformation. In R. Barnett and N. Jackson (eds), *Ecologies for Learning and Practice: Emerging Ideas, Sightings and Possibilities*. Abingdon: Routledge. pp. 46–60.

Scheeres, H., Solomon, N., Boud, D. and Rooney, D. (2010). When is it okay to learn at work? The learning work of organisational practices. *Journal of Workplace Learning*, 22(1&2): 13–26.

Schön, D. (1987) *Educating the Reflective Practitioner*. San Francisco: Jossey-Bass.

Scott, H. (2004) Are nurses 'too clever to care' and 'too posh to wash'? *British Journal of Nursing*, 13(10): 582.

Shaw, M. (1993) The discipline of nursing: historical roots, current perspectives, future directions. *Journal of Advanced Nursing*, 18(10): 1651–1656.

Smeby, J.-C., and Vågan, A. (2008a) Recontextualising professional knowledge: newly qualified nurses and physicians. *Journal of Education and Work*, 21(2): 159–173.

Smeby, J.-C. and Vågan, A. (2008b) Caught in the science trap? A case study of the relationship between nurses and 'their' science. In J. Välimaa and O.-H. Ylijoki (eds), *Cultural Perspectives on Higher Education*. New York: Springer. pp. 127–141.

Smith, J. P. (1994) *Models, Theories and Concepts*. Oxford: Blackwell.

Smith, P. A. (2013) Counter the scape-goating and show the public you still care. 11 February 2013. Retrieved from: www.nursingtimes.net/nursing-practice/clinical-zones/practice-nursing/counter-the-scapegoating-and-show-the-public-you-still-care/5054842.article

Smith, P. and Allan, H. T. (2010) We should be able to bear our patients in our teaching in some way: theoretical perspectives on how nurse teachers manage their emotions to negotiate the split between education and caring practice. *Nurse Education Today*, 30(3): 218–223.

Smith, P. A. and Allan, H. T. (2016) Women's work. In H. T. Allan, D. Kelly, P. Smith and M. Traynor (eds), *Understanding Sociology in Nursing*. London: Sage. pp. 55–78.

Smith, P. M., Corso, L. N. and Cobb, N. (2010) The perennial struggle to find clinical placement opportunities: a Canadian national survey. *Nurse Education Today*, 30(8): 798–803.

Smith, P., MacKintosh, M. M., Ross, F., Clayton, J., Price, L., Christian, S., Byng, R. and Allan, H. T. (2012) Financial and clinical risk in health care reform: a view from below. *Journal of Health Services Research Policy*, 17(Suppl 2): 11–17.

Solomon, N., Boud, D. and Rooney, D. (2006) The in-between: exposing everyday learning at work. *International Journal of Lifelong Education*, 25(1): 3–13.

Spitzer, A. and Perrenoud, B. (2006) Reforms in nursing education across Western Europe: from agenda to practice. *Journal of Professional Nursing*, 22(3): 150–161.

Spouse, J. (1998) Scaffolding student learning in clinical practice. *Nurse Education Today*, 18: 259–266.

Spouse, J. (2001a) Work-based learning in health care environments. *Nurse Education in Practice*, 1(1): 12–18.

Spouse, J. (2001b) Bridging theory and practice in the supervisory relationship: a sociocultural perspective. *Journal of Advanced Nursing*, 33(4): 512–522.

Street, A. F. (1992) *Inside Nursing: A Critical Ethnography of Clinical Nursing Practice*. New York: State University of New York.

Sveningsson, S. and Alvesson, M. (2003) Managing managerial identities: organizational fragmentation, discourse and identity struggle. *Human Relations*, 56(10): 1163–1193.

Taylor, M. and Evans, K. (2009) Formal and informal training for workers with low literacy: constructing an international dialogue between Canada and the UK. *Journal of Adult and Continuing Education*, 9: 37–52.

ten Hoeve, Y., Jansen, G. and Roodbol, P. (2013) The nursing profession: public image, self-concept and professional identity. A discussion paper. *Journal of Advanced Nursing*, 70(2): 295–309.

The Open University (2018) *Tackling the Nursing Shortage*. Milton Keynes: Open University Press.

Thomas, S. (2013) Using the principles of Vygotsky in the home environment: a health visitor's perspective for under-fives. *Journal of Health Visiting*, 1(7): 380–383.

Trevithick, C. (2013) *A research study to analyse the perceived leadership development needs of Board nurses in Clinical Commissioning Groups in light of the Health and Social Care Act 2012, in order to develop the Board nurse role*. Unpublished MA thesis. De Montfort University. September 2013.

United Kingdom Central Council for Nursing, Midwifery and Health Visiting (1986) *Project 2000: A New Preparation for Practice*. London: UKCC.

Vähäsantanen, K., Hökkä, P., Paloniemi, S., Herranen, S. and Eteläpelto, A. (2017) Professional learning and agency in an identity coaching programme. *Professional Development in Education*, 43(4): 514–536.

Van Gennep, A. (1960 [1909]) *Rites of Passage (Les rites de passage)*. trans. M. B. Vizedom and G. L. Caffee. Chicago: The University of Chicago Press.

van Oers, B. (1998) The fallacy of decontextualisation. *Mind, Culture and Activity*, 5(2): 143–152.

Vygotsky, L. and Luria, A. (1930) Tool and symbol in child development. In R. Van der Veer and J. Valsiner (eds), *The Vygotsky Reader*. Oxford: Blackwell. pp. 99–174.

Walani, S. (2015) Global migration of internationally educated nurses: experiences of employment discrimination. *International Journal of Africa Nursing Sciences*, 3: 65–70.

Walby, S., Greenwell, J., MacKay, L. and Soothill, K. (1994) *Medicine and Nursing Professionals in a Changing Health Service*. London: Sage.

Watson, J. (1979) *Nursing: The Philosophy and Science of Caring*. New York: Little, Brown and Co.

Watson, J. (1988) *Nursing: Human Science and Human Care*. New York: Appleton-Century-Croft.

Watson, T. J. (2008) Managing identity: identity work, personal predicaments and structural circumstances. *Organization*, 15(1): 121–143.

West, M. (2004) *Effective Teamwork: Practical Lessons from Organisational Research*. Oxford: Blackwell.

West, M., Brodbeck, F. and Richter, A. (2004) Does the 'romance of teams' exist? The effectiveness of teams in experimental and field settings. *Journal of Occupational and Organisational Psychology*, 77: 467–473.

Weydt, A. (2010). Developing delegation skills. *The Online Journal of Issues in Nursing*, 15(2). Retrieved from: https://ojin.nursingworld.org/MainMenuCategories/ANAMarketplace/ANAPeriodicals/OJIN/TableofContents/Vol152010/No2May2010/Delegation-Skills.html

Whitehead, B., Owen, P. et al. (2013) Supporting newly qualified nurses in the UK: a systematic literature review. *Nurse Education Today*, 33: 370–377.

Wilkinson, G. and Miers, M. (1999) *Power and Nursing Practice*. Basingstoke: Macmillan.

Willetts, G. and Clarke, D. (2014) Constructing nurses' professional identity through social identity theory. *International Journal of Nursing Practice*, 20(2): 164–169.

Wimpenny, P. (2002) The meaning of models of nursing to practicing nurses. *Journal of Advanced Nursing*, 40(3): 346–354.

Yancey, N. R. (2015) Why teach nursing theory? *Nursing Science Quarterly*, 28(4): 274–278.

Index

Activities of Daily Living (ADL) model 3–4
adaptive recontextualisation 75–7, 87–8, 93–4, 122–4, 142
Advanced Nurse Practice (ACP) 21
aesthetic learning 29, 34
agency
   nurses 104–6, 109–10, 128, 131–2, 142–4, 146, 148, 155
   patient 18, 22, 23
Allmark, P. 34, 158
apprenticeship model 3, 14, 21, 27, 147

Barnett, R. 6, 12, 141–2, 152, 153
Benner, P. 156
Benson, A. 149
Bernstein, B. B. 37
biomedical model 3
biomedicine 17, 52
blood pressure measurement 29, 59, 74
Bradshaw, A. 7
Brammer, J. D. 148, 149–50
BSc Nurse Practitioner 85
bullying 18, 121

Canales, M. 103, 133, 141
capitalism 15
Carper, B. 33
Carr, W. 156
Chinn, P. 136–7
Chisholm, L. 28
climate crisis 22, 23
Clinical Commissioning Groups (CCGs) 17–18
   see also governing body nurses (GBN) (study 5)
clinical placements see workplace
clinical role-modelling 149
codification 38
cognitive apprenticeship model 147
commissioning board 17, 54
commissioning nurses see governing body nurses (GBN) (study 5)
communities of practice 27
Compassion in Practice (CiP) 8, 19
competence-based learning 58
constructivism 30
content recontextualisation 37–8, 40–1, 61
continuous professional development 57, 59, 101, 128, 155
Cousin, G. 104

covert medication policy 98
Covid-19 pandemic 14, 131, 142–3, 158
critical reflection 6, 32, 156
critical theory 32
Crowley, D. M. 8, 132–3

de-bordering 28
Delegate (study 2) 6, 10, 47–50, 131, 135, 144, 149
   learner recontextualisation 116, 125
   workplace recontextualisation 62–80
Dewey, John 30–1
Dickoff, J. 133
disintegrated learning 42, 142, 145, 146–50, 154
district nurse consultants 114–15
Donaldson, S. K. 8, 132–3
Drevdahl, D. 103, 133, 141

ecologies of learning approach 11–12, 80, 131, 146, 152–4, 159
economic crisis 17
emancipatory knowledge 31–2, 130
Emirbayer, M. 104
emotional learning 34
empirical knowledge 29, 34, 63
empiricism 29, 33, 136–7
enacted knowledge 134, 143
   learner recontextualisation 104, 107–8, 120–2
   workplace recontextualisation 62, 68, 74, 93
ENRIP study 21
environment 22, 23
Eraut, Michael 30, 31–2
ethical learning 29, 34
evidence-based approaches 29, 33, 139
Expert Patients Programme 18

Fabricius, J. 155
Fawcett, J. 22, 157
Fealy, G. M. 140, 147, 156
fertility nursing (study 4) 10, 52–3, 131, 144, 149
   identity 141
   learner recontextualisation 109–10, 120, 124–5
   workplace recontextualisation 81–101
   see also IVF clinics
figured worlds 104
Fitness for Practice (F4P) 21
Francisco, S. 147
Francis Report 7, 19–20, 24, 54

gender
  health inequalities 15
  NHS employees 17
  nursing origins 18–19
  pay gap 17
Gill, D. 104
governing body nurses (GBN) (study 5) 10,
    53–5, 81–101, 131, 133, 141, 144, 149
  workplace recontextualisation 81–101
GP contracts 18
gradual release 134, 143
  learner recontextualisation 107, 118–20
  workplace recontextualisation 61, 67, 68,
    71–3, 93
grand theories 1–2, 4, 7, 11, 19, 33, 130,
    133–40, 145, 156

healthcare assistants (HCAs) 151
  Delegate study 47–50
  learner recontextualisation 108–10, 125
  workplace recontextualisation 63, 66–7, 69,
    72, 74
health inequalities 15–16
Health and Social Care Act 17
Heggen, K. 138
Henderson, V. 22, 31
hierarchies of evidence 139
Hökkä, P. K. 104, 105, 106, 155
Holland, D. 104

idealism 6, 8
identity *see* professional identity
infant mortality rate 15
informal learning 27, 30
integrating learning 111–12
internal milieu 82, 96
International Council of Nurses (ICN) 22–3
interpretation acts
  learner recontextualisation 112–13
  workplace recontextualisation 62–5,
    82–3, 86
interpretative-constructionist approach 33
intuitive knowledge 32
IVF clinics 60
  see also fertility nursing

Jackson, D. 146
Jackson, N. 6, 12, 141–2, 152, 153
James, P. 133
Jensen, K. 139
journeypersons 148
Judge Report 20

Kersh, N. 102, 103
Kikuchi, J. F. 133
Kira, M. 142
Kitson, A. 139–40
know-how 9, 35–6, 38, 79, 130

knowledge
  development 32–3, 36
  flows 37
  hierarchy 33, 34, 35
  transfer 31–2, 36, 43
  ways of knowing 33–6
  see also recontextualisation
know-that knowledge 9, 35–6, 38, 68, 79, 130
Kramer, M. K. 136–7

Lahn, L. 139
Laiho, A. 137, 138
Land, R. 150–1
Latter, S. 149
Lave, J. 148
Lawler, J. A. 34, 54
Leadership for Learning (study 1) 10, 45–7,
    131, 144, 149
  learner recontextualisation 117–18
  workplace recontextualisation 67–8, 75–6,
    78–80
learner recontextualisation (LR) 11, 37, 40–1,
    58, 102–28, 132, 134, 143–4, 146, 151,
    153, 155, 158
learning conversation approach 40, 42, 62, 67,
    93, 106, 108, 120
learning as doing 31
Leininger, M. 4, 7, 9
life expectancy 15
lifelong learning 11, 57–9, 102–3, 108, 127,
    132, 134, 143, 145, 147, 153, 155
liminality 11, 104, 145, 150–2
Logan, W. 3–4
long-term conditions *see PEGI* study
    (study 3)

McBride, A. B. 141
McKenna, H. 2, 9, 11, 24, 33, 35–6, 42, 130,
    133, 135–6, 143
managerialism 17, 18, 53–4
Manley, K. 8, 25, 36, 130, 135, 143
Mannix, J. 146
marketisation 18
May, Theresa 18
medical point of view 64
mental health teams (study 3) 132
  workplace recontextualisation 81–101
mentors and supervisors 27, 41, 132, 147–50
  feedback 62
  learner recontextualisation 119–21
  relationship 30
  workplace recontextualisation 62–3, 67–8,
    76–7
Menzies-Lyth, I. E. P. 155
meta-cognitive strategies 41, 58, 103
mid-range theories 1, 2, 11, 135–6, 145, 157
migrant workforce 19, 105–6, 127
Mische, A. 104

modified early warning score (MEWS) 61
Mothers and Babies: Reducing Risk through
	Audits and Confidential Enquiries across
	the UK (MBRRACE-UK) 15

new knowledge enactment *see* enacted
	knowledge
newly qualified nurses (NQNs) 132, 149
	agency 142
	Delegate study 47–50
	identity 141
	learner recontextualisation 108–12, 116–27
	liminality 150, 151
	workplace recontextualisation 63–79
	see also Delegate (study 2); *Leadership for
		Learning* (study 1)
Nightingale, Florence 3, 20, 21
nursing assistants 21
Nursing and Midwifery Council (NMC) 20, 21,
	23, 24, 147, 148, 157

occupational therapists 97–8, 113–15, 130
online learning 158
oppressive power structures 32

pathophysiology 29
patient agency 18, 22, 23
patient choice 18
patient observations 61
patient relationship 31, 94
patient safety culture 19–20
Patient's Charter 18
patient wellbeing 87–8
Pawson, R. 51
pedagogic recontextualisation 37, 38–9,
	40–1, 61
peer learning groups 63
PEGI study (study 3) 10, 51–2, 87–8, 130, 131,
	132, 144
	learner recontextualisation 112–13
	workplace recontextualisation 81–101
Peplau, H. 7, 31
personal knowledge 31
personal learning 34
person-centred theory 11, 24–5, 130, 135, 140, 143
personhood and autonomy 22–3
'positive borderlessness' 28
post-positivism 29, 33
post-traumatic stress disorders 131
practice architecture approaches 147, 148
pressure care 65–6
primary care 18, 87–8, 93, 113, 133, 141
primary care trusts (PCTs) 52, 99
prior learning 40, 48, 103, 107, 127, 132, 144
procedural knowledge 68, 79, 130
process knowledge 31
productive recontextualisation 77–9, 95–100,
	124–6, 142

professional identity 103–4, 106, 108, 115, 133,
	141–3
	liminality 150, 152
Project 2000 4, 20–1, 121
propositional knowledge 31
psychodynamic approach 7, 124, 155

Quinlan, K. 147

race
	health inequalities 15
	nursing origins 18
	pay gap 17
	racism 19
rationalism 29, 33
realism 6, 8
recontextualisation 6, 8, 10–12, 24, 28, 30,
	36–43
	see also content recontextualisation; learner
		recontextualisation; pedagogic
		recontextualisation; workplace
		recontextualisation
reflection 36, 137, 156
	learner recontextualisation 104, 112
	workplace recontextualisation 62, 78–9
reflection-in-action 32, 104
reflection-on-action 31, 32
reification 7
religion, nursing origins 18
resilience 101, 127, 130, 143, 155
Richardson, B. 54, 55
Rogers, B. 159
role modelling 68
Rolfe, G. 31
Roper, N. 3–4
routines 143
	learner recontextualisation 104
	workplace recontextualisation 61, 64, 69, 74
Ruoholinna, T. 137, 138

Savin-Baden, M. 150, 151, 152
Schön, D. 33–4
'seeing the whole' 111–15
self-care 22, 23, 24
self-reflection 104
service redesign 85, 87, 89, 99
service user reference groups (SURGs) 52
Shape of Caring 20
'shared purpose' 25
Shaw, M. 14
Simmons, H. 133
simulations 31
situated learning 30, 41
skills-based teaching 137, 140, 152
Smith, J. P. 136
social changes 9, 13–24
social class 15, 19
social conservatism 152

social constructivism 30
Song, Y. 147
spatial associations 103, 112, 127, 132
Spouse, J. 146
Standards Framework for Nursing and
    Midwifery Education 147
Standards for Supervision and Assessment 148
stereotypes 18–19
structuration 105–6
student nurses 132
    clinical placements 146–7
    Covid-19 pandemic 142–3
    identity 141
    inclusion 27
    Leadership for Learning study 45–7
    see also Delegate (study 2); *Leadership for*
        Learning (study 1)
study 1 *see Leadership for Learning* (study 1)
study 2 *see* Delegate (study 2)
study 3 *see PEGI* study (study 3)
study 4 *see* fertility nursing (study 4)
study 5 *see* governing body nurses (GBN) (study 5)

tacit knowledge 31, 35, 40, 130, 132
    learner recontextualisation 103
    workplace recontextualisation 63, 68, 79
task allocation 47, 137
technology 21
theory–practice gap 6–7, 36, 41–3, 130, 137–9,
    147, 155–6
theory–practice split 6–7, 56, 103, 127–8, 130,
    132, 137–9, 147, 152, 156
Tierney, A. 3–4
Tilley, N. 51

time management skills 72–3
time/predictability 134, 143
    learner recontextualisation 107, 116–18
    workplace recontextualisation 61–2,
        68–71, 92
Traynor, Michael 19

Vähäsantanen, K. 142
values-based recruitment (VBR) 20
Valuing and Recognising the Talents of a
    Diverse Healthcare Workforce 105–6
van Gennep, A. 150
van Oers, B. 37, 39
Vygotsky, Lev 30, 147

ward culture 49, 115
ward managers (WM) 65–7, 70, 72–3,
    118–19, 149
ward teams 27, 111, 142
Watson, J. 4, 7
Watson, T. J. 141
Wenger, E. 148
Willis Commission 20
Winterbourne View of learning disability 19
workplace
    learning 26–8, 146–7, 157–8
    reorganisation 89–91, 114
    as a whole 111–15
workplace recontextualisation (WR) 37, 39,
    40–1, 143, 146, 151, 153, 155, 158
    experienced nurses 81–101
    theorising in practice 10, 57–101

zone of proximal development (ZPD) 30, 148